Healthcare Simulation in Practice

Mark Hellaby

Other books from M&K include:

Mentorship in Healthcare
ISBN: 9781905539703

The ECG Workbook 2/e
ISBN: 9781905539772

Routine Blood Results Explained 3/e
ISBN: 9781905539888

Practical Aspects of ECG Recording
ISBN: 9781905539307

Blood Results in Clinical Practice
ISBN: 9781905539734

Ward Based Critical Care
ISBN: 9781905539031

Self assessment in Axial Skeleton Musculoskeletal Trauma X-rays
ISBN: 9781905539475

Self assessment in Paediatric Musculoskeletal Trauma X-rays
ISBN: 9781905539345

Healthcare Simulation in Practice

Mark Hellaby

Healthcare Simulation in Practice

Mark Hellaby

ISBN: 9781905539-56-7

First published 2013

British Library Cataloguing in Publication Data

A catalogue record for this book is available from the British Library

Notice

Clinical practice and medical knowledge constantly evolve. Standard safety precautions must be followed, but, as knowledge is broadened by research, changes in practice, treatment and drug therapy may become necessary or appropriate. Readers must check the most current product information provided by the manufacturer of each drug to be administered and verify the dosages and correct administration, as well as contraindications. It is the responsibility of the practitioner, utilising the experience and knowledge of the patient, to determine dosages and the best treatment for each individual patient. Any brands mentioned in this book are as examples only and are not endorsed by the publisher. Neither the publisher nor the authors assume any liability for any injury and/or damage to persons or property arising from this publication.

To contact M&K Publishing write to:

M&K Update Ltd · The Old Bakery · St. John's Street

Keswick · Cumbria CA12 5AS

Tel: 01768 773030 · Fax: 01768 781099

publishing@mkupdate.co.uk

www.mkupdate.co.uk

Designed and typeset by Mary Blood

Printed in England by H&H Reeds, Penrith

Contents

Preface

This book is intended as a resource for all those involved in undergraduate and postgraduate simulation-based education, whether for uni-professional or multi-professional learners. Although it is primarily directed at those using simulation within a hospital or practice environment, I hope it will also be a useful resource for simulation activities within other healthcare settings, higher education institutions and voluntary organisations.

Most people have heard of healthcare simulation and some agree that simulation is a good thing and we need more of it. However, there is often some confusion about what the term 'simulation' actually means, and what simulation can and can't achieve.

In fact, simulation is being used more and more in hospital settings. It is no longer unusual for organisations to have a formal established area where simulated learning sessions can be run. Quite often, learners may in addition have access to simulation in various clinical practice areas. Many of the recommendations of the recent Francis report (Francis 2013) can be implemented at an organisational level using a variety of simulation initiatives. There is now an opportunity for simulation to change from merely being a reactive process (in which a targeted group prepares for a particular type of incident by using a single simulation as an isolated event) to a proactive process (in which repeated simulations allow development of the entire workforce over a period of time and identify organisational and cultural issues). To achieve this change, simulation facilitators need to work together in a coordinated, evidence-based manner, across organisational, departmental and regional barriers, actively involving local higher educational institutions and stakeholders in a collaborative way.

If simulation is not facilitated using sound educational practice, facilitators risk failing the learners they are trying to help and tarnishing the reputation of simulation. The stages in which each session is developed, planned, validated, facilitated and evaluated need to be robust and supported by a trained faculty. Too often, the scenario is the starting point for planning, and the learning outcomes happen by chance. There is an over-reliance on the scenario, and a lack of appreciation of the importance of the debriefing period, when the real learning and change in practice may be achieved.

The clinical course of the scenario must be realistic and peer-reviewed, and all scenarios need to demonstrate validity and reliability. There should be a robust quality assurance process embedded in every step of the simulation event. This will demonstrate that simulation is being used effectively and appropriately. It will also show that the simulation is offering value for money and is ultimately improving patient care. More and more individuals and organisations are using simulation, although concern has been expressed about the level of faculty education of those involved in the simulation process (McGaghie *et al.* 2010). The main aim of this book is to fill this gap, by giving simulation facilitators a deeper understanding of the process they are using.

The Department of Health (DH) has published guidance on technology-enhanced learning, which includes simulation. The Framework of Technology Enhanced Learning (DH 2011) identifies six key principles that technology-enhanced learning should conform to. It should:

- Be patient-centred
- Be educationally coherent
- Be innovative and evidence-based
- Deliver high-quality educational outcomes
- Deliver value for money
- Ensure equity of access and quality of provision.

In this book, the focus is on the simulation process as a whole, rather than the details of how particular simulations are delivered. This is deliberate because it allows the reader to gain an overview of the steps required to achieve educational goals, whether by using a manikin or a faculty member as an actor and whatever equipment is used. The book reflects simulation practice within secondary healthcare organisations in the context of relevant scenarios. The theory of simulation is also transferable to other healthcare domains, such as primary healthcare, mental health, learning disability and pre-hospital care settings. Although the specific scenario content will change, the basic structure of the simulation process that is described will not.

I have written this book for staff working within organisations that are currently using or wish to use simulation as a learning tool. It is very much an introduction. Ultimately, the real learning will occur through putting it all into practice, leading to increased confidence and competence.

I have deliberately included chapters on simulation run within actual clinical practice areas, in-situ training and simulation in a dedicated formal simulation learning area. There is no suggestion that simulation in a practice setting is more or less beneficial than simulation in a dedicated learning environment. Indeed, each method has pros and cons. They can identify different issues, and can be used to focus on different learning outcomes or to reinforce each other in a complementary manner.

I have enjoyed facilitating and planning simulation sessions for many years – particularly seeing the engagement and enthusiasm of learners when enlightenment suddenly strikes. I hope this book will help other facilitators to experience this sense of satisfaction too.

References

Department of Health (2011). *A Framework for Technology Enhanced Learning*. London: HMSO.

Francis, R. (2013). *Report of the Mid Staffordshire NHS Foundation Trust Public Inquiry*. London: HMSO.

McGaghie, W.C., Issenberg, S.B., Petrusa, E.R. & Scalese, R.J. (2010). A critical review of simulation-based medical education research: 2003–2009. *Medical Education*. **44**, 50–63.

About the Author

Mark Hellaby M. Ed., BSc (Hons), RODP, FHEA, MCODP
NHS NorthWest Simulation Network Manager
ASPiH/Higher Education Academy Simulation Development Officer (SDO)
Professional Editor, *Technic: The Journal of Operating Department Practice*

Mark Hellaby is the North West Simulation Education Network Manager, with a strong interest in simulation, human factors, patient safety and research on effectiveness and outcomes of simulation. He has a Masters Degree in professional education and is an Operating Department Practitioner by background.

Having worked in the health service for over 20 years he has been involved in simulation both within critical care areas and also pre-hospital medicine. Since 2008 he has worked full time within an NHS organisation as a Simulation/Clinical Skills facilitator and was responsible for establishing simulation, in particular for undergraduate medical and the trust foundation doctors. In this role he developed multi-professional in-situ simulation sessions as well as learning sessions in a dedicated simulation area.

Mark's current role with the network is primarily involved in increasing capability and capacity of simulation throughout the north west of England in both the NHS and partner academic organisations. He has also been appointed as the NW Simulation Development Officer for the Association of Simulation in Practice in Healthcare (ASPiH)/Higher Education Academy (HEA) project.

Chapter 1

What is simulation?

Key points

- The terms simulation and fidelity are often misused and misunderstood
- There is often a fixation on the scenario and specifically the manikin
- Simulation is a process that includes numerous steps
- The goal of any simulation event should be effective learning and benefit to patient care and safety
- There is a need for facilitators to be educated and their skills developed in simulation theory and debriefing skills
- Facilitators need an awareness of how healthcare errors are caused and propagated

Over the last 50 years (DH 2011), there has been considerable interest in the use of simulation for healthcare education. Simulation was originally restricted to regional simulation centres for specific identified learners, often as a one-off event. Often the simulation was designed to teach clinical procedures. However, there is currently an explosion in simulation use within many different healthcare organisations. This chapter will look at what is understood by the term simulation. It will briefly mention the two main educational theories linked to simulation and discuss the concept of fidelity and realism. The different areas of simulation will be introduced and finally the subject of healthcare error will be mentioned.

The old medical education approach of 'see one, do one, teach one' (whilst learning on actual patients) has been described as inappropriate for the twenty-first century (Donaldson 2009) and has raised ethical questions about the use of patients as a training resource (Issenberg & Scalese 2008). Meanwhile, the reduction in teaching time and practice placements has increased the need for high-quality education. As the focus has shifted from the apprenticeship model to an outcome-based approach, simulation has been proposed as an ideal method of assessing competence.

Simulation can also be used to enhance the ad hoc nature of practice education and give all learners a standardised experience of rarer cases and incidents. Performing simulations in-situ, in the actual practice environment, allows for training of the extended team, including individuals who would not normally be the focus of more formal training. It has been found that such sessions can help detect organisational system-based risks in the clinical environment and reduce patient and institutional risk (Yajamanyam *et al.* 2012). Indeed, while serving as Chief Medical Officer, Sir Liam Donaldson called for simulation-based training to be fully integrated, resourced and supported by a skilled faculty to enable high-quality training (Donaldson 2009).

What is simulation?

One cannot describe how to fund, evaluate or train people to use simulation without first defining it. The prevailing confusion about the meaning of simulation is partly due to the lack of clear national simulation standards and strategies. There are also many different reasons that people may have for running simulations. The aim may be to recreate a rare or unfamiliar event so that individuals can develop experiential learning and become familiar with it. Alternatively, trainers may choose an event and repeat it a number of times so that students can learn through deliberate practice; or they may take a routine clinical event but focus on the team working and communication aspects, in an attempt to develop those particular skills. Simulation is a word that is often used and equally often misunderstood. It can actually involve a variety of different technologies and equipment (see Table 1.1, page 7).

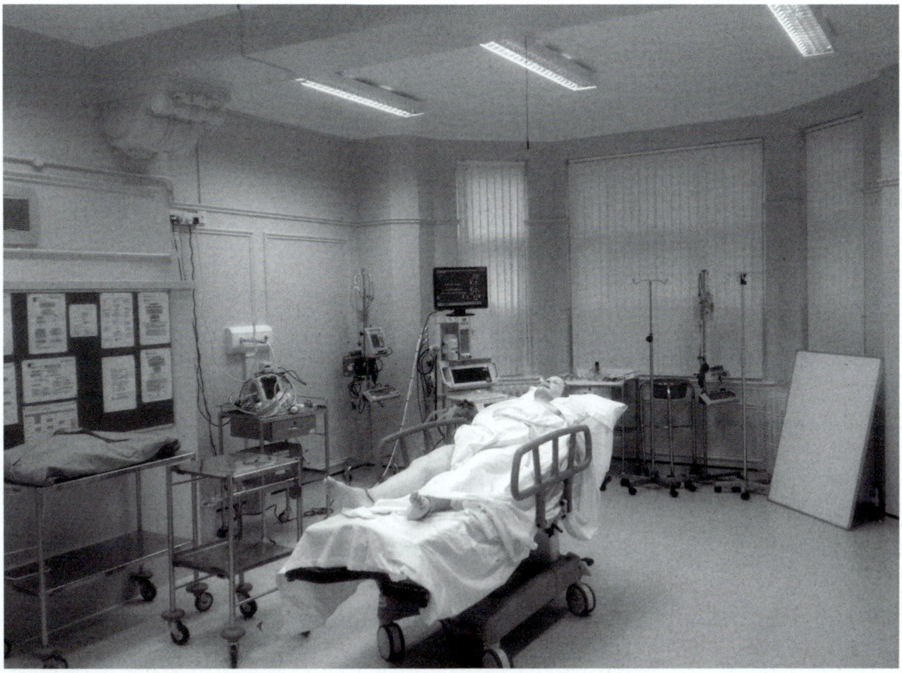

Figure 1.1
This is most people's idea of healthcare simulation (a manikin in the Simulation Centre at North Manchester General Hospital) but it is by no means the only possible modality.

Part of the problem with establishing what is meant by simulation is the fact that people get fixated on the scenario (and specifically the manikin) and don't always appreciate that simulation is a process with many interlinked stages that starts long before the simulation session and should continue far beyond it. David Gaba makes this point when he says 'simulation is a technique, not a technology' (Gaba 2004). A systematic review from the Best Evidence Medical Education (BEME) Collaboration identified 10 features that facilitators should be aware of and adopt when using simulation (Issenberg *et al.* 2005):

1. Feedback
2. Repetitive practice
3. Range of difficulty levels
4. Multiple learning strategies
5. Clinical variation
6. Controlled environment
7. Individualised learning
8. Defined outcomes/benchmarks
9. Simulation validity/realism
10. Curriculum integration.

Throughout this book, simulation is simply described as an attempt to 'recreate a real life task, event or experience, providing a safe learning environment, for the acquisition of skills, knowledge, attitudes and behaviors' (MacKinnon 2011). Note that this definition is deliberately broad, in order to be as inclusive as possible of all the different modalities of simulation. Actual patients have been included as a simulation modality, as there are times when patients are selected for training wards staffed by students or used in clinical examination training.

Simulation is often initially viewed as a tool to teach clinical procedures. However, the above definition demonstrates that it can be used not only to develop knowledge and skills but also to focus on attitudes, ways of behaving and their development. Thus, the same scenario can be used for a number of different learning outcomes. In recent years, there has been considerable interest in the use of simulation for inter-professional education, with a particular focus on patient safety (Gough *et al.* 2012). Innovative simulation sessions are increasingly being used to develop a greater awareness of how to recognise and prevent patient harm incidents and the human factors that can contribute to them.

Educational theories and simulation

The two main educational theories associated with simulation-based education are experiential learning (constructivism) and deliberate practice (behaviourism). David Kolb (1983) described the experiential learning cycle and recognised that learners have preferred learning styles. He described a cycle, where a learner experiences an event (concrete experience), then reflects on the event (reflective observation), forms new views (abstract conceptualisation) and finally puts these views into practice (active experimentation). Peter Honey and Alan Mumford (Honey & Mumford 1982) adapted Kolb's experiential model and assigned four different learning styles to the cycle: activist (concrete experience), reflector (reflective observation), theorist (abstract conceptualisation) and pragmatist (active experimentation). They then developed a questionnaire to identify individuals' learning style(s), based on the assumption that every learner has a preferred style or styles.

Each simulated learning event has elements that engage with these different learning styles, whether in the scenario, debriefing or subsequent scenario where learning is put into action. Experiential learning is described as a form of constructivism, in which learners construct their understanding of the world through their interaction with it, by means of a process of assimilation and accommodation (Bradley & Postlethwaite 2003). The central tenet of constructivism is that learning is an active process in which the lecturer acts as a guide or facilitator (Tam 2000). Because simulation is now recognised as taking a constructivist approach, we refer to those who guide the scenario or debriefing as facilitators.

Deliberate practice, in which the learner repeats a task and receives rigorous assessment and specific feedback, aims to achieve better skills performance (Duvivier *et al.* 2011), which becomes fluent and instinctive (Weller *et al.* 2012). Often, the task is a cognitive or psychomotor one (Grant 2012). There is also an emphasis on motivation and feedback (Castanelli 2009), which aligns it more to behaviouristic theory, where a positive behaviour is rewarded and any action is a learnt behaviour.

Fidelity and simulation

Fidelity (in relation to simulation) is another word that is often misused or not fully understood. It is also multi-dimensional (Beaubien & Baker 2004) and originates from descriptions of aircraft flight simulators. The term fidelity refers to how closely the simulation imitates the real-life event. Whilst imitation is the aim, it is not clear what level of fidelity is required to achieve authenticity (Bland *et al.* 2011).

As already stated, a simulation requires far more than just a manikin. Whilst simulation hardware is part of the process, it is by no means the whole story. With aircraft simulators, the air crew interact directly with technology and the same equipment can therefore be used in a simulator to recreate a very realistic cockpit environment. However, healthcare staff interact with people (not just equipment), and a manikin is never a perfect representation of a patient. Manikins may be described as low fidelity (for instance, a part task trainer such as a cannulation arm), medium fidelity (for example, a resuscitation manikin, perhaps with ECG and other physical parameters) and finally high fidelity (such as the very realistic human patient simulators, which can breathe, blink, sweat and react physiologically to drugs and events). As we have seen, it is not just the fidelity of the manikin that gives a simulation defined fidelity. Yet the two are often equated in research and published literature. Does a low-fidelity manikin only allow a low-fidelity simulation? Does a high-fidelity manikin always ensure a high-fidelity simulation? The answer is 'Clearly not'.

Equipment, environment and psychology can also have varying degrees of fidelity. For instance, how far does the simulation mirror the actual environment and equipment the learner would normally work with (Berragan 2011)? Environmental fidelity includes the physical layout, the provision of other supporting equipment, and the test results that would normally be available. Psychological fidelity involves the extent to which learners believe in the scenario and whether they feel it is a realistic equivalent to an actual clinical episode.

I have to say, because of the misuse, confusion and inconsistency surrounding the term 'fidelity', it is not a word I often use. Gaba (2004) and others have suggested terms that better describe elements of a simulated event but these are not in widespread use.

Table 1.1: **Different types of simulation**

Type of simulation	Example
Online virtual simulation	Virtual central line training course
Simulation using part task trainers	Cannulation arm, airway head
Simulation using standardised patients or actors	Breaking bad news, communication training
Human patient simulation	Low, medium and high fidelity patient simulators
Actual patient simulation	Training ward
Virtual world simulation	Second Life

Realism and simulation

True immersive simulation occurs when we recreate the complete environment so accurately that learners cannot distinguish it from reality. It is unusual to achieve this completely within a healthcare setting (Hotchkiss *et al.* 2002). This is partly because of the limitations of the equipment used and also because the learners usually know that they are attending a simulation. The aim is to create a safe environment in which students are permitted to make errors. However, if the scenario is *too realistic*, students may feel over-anxious and concerned about doing harm, and learning could be prevented. Alinier (2010) states that the right balance needs to be achieved between realism and added value for the participants' educational experience. He also refers to the article by Peter Dieckmann and colleagues, which stated that it is not uniformly the case that greater realism helps to achieve better educational goals (Dieckmann *et al.* 2007). Because the learners are aware that it is a simulation and not a real patient, there is an initial requirement to buy in (or participate in) the simulation. However, once the scenario has started, they often get drawn into the situation and react more and more as they would in practice.

It should also be remembered that the more technically realistic the scenario, the more maintenance and repair it will often require. This may limit the number of facilitators who are able to use it, and could even mean that the institution has to employ a designated technician to maintain the simulation equipment. In addition, more time may be required to prepare the scenario before using it on each occasion.

Assessment and simulation

Simulation always involves a degree of assessment. Without this, it is not possible to identify how learners have deviated from the expected norm, give them feedback about their performance or assess how effective the session was. Fortunately, it is still more common for simulation to be used as part of a formative session, with feedback given in the form of a debriefing, as opposed to a summative, exam-type session with a pass/fail result.

The common exception to this rule is resuscitation training, where there is often some type of summative assessment during the session. The integral use of simulation as an assessment tool (for both formative and summative purposes) requires facilitators to confirm that simulation sessions are a valid, reliable and appropriate tool for this type of training.

Value for money?

We also need to assess whether simulation offers value for money. As we have seen, simulation comes at a high price – because of the relatively high capital equipment costs and also because of the high ratio of facilitators to learners. In view of this, we need to be sure that each planned session is not only best suited to simulation but also that we are making the most effective use of resources. For instance, using an expensive, high-fidelity human patient simulator to practise cannulation is not a sensible use of resources.

Ideally, an identified person or group should take an overview of simulation across the organisation. As interest in simulation increases, there will often be a push from both educators and senior managers to use simulation in more and more sessions. If we are not careful, this can easily lead to 'simulation for simulation's sake', rather than consciously choosing to use simulation because of its relevance and appropriateness in providing the relevant learning outcomes.

Simulation should also be seen as a part of a blended approach to learning, rather than a stand-alone strategy (DH 2011). It should reinforce and reflect existing skills, knowledge and behaviours as well as developing new ones. Within the NHS, this means that multiple providers should be working together so that common messages are being reinforced across different departments and professions. Simulation sessions will also often be run in collaboration with local higher education institutions to guarantee that the training reflects the needs of undergraduate learners as well.

The elements of simulation

Every simulation requires a faculty or set of facilitators, a scenario and a group of learners.

The simulation faculty

The facilitators who come together to form the simulation faculty need to be trained in the effective use of simulation-based education (Issenberg 2006). This is not only in order to fulfil the requirement for clinical credibility but also to ensure that they have an understanding of the application, limitation and practicalities of using simulation. Simulation knowledge typically tends to be gained through trial and error. It is not standardised and can therefore have variable effectiveness. McGaghie and colleagues (2010) suggested that there was a lack of any process to educate, evaluate and certify faculty involved in healthcare simulation, while Issenberg *et al.* discussed the role of the healthcare educator for simulation-based training as an information provider, role model, facilitator, assessor, planner and resource developer (Issenberg 2006).

It is always essential to provide a safe environment and work *with* the learners, as opposed to telling them or lecturing them. This means treating learners as individual adults, understanding that they have previously acquired knowledge and realising how best they can put the knowledge they gain into practice (Knowles 1980). The phrase 'safe environment' will be mentioned several times throughout this book. It should also be reinforced several times throughout each session to reassure and explain the process to the learners and to get them to participate fully in both the scenario and the debriefing session. Only if learners feel free to explain their thought processes can facilitators gain a real understanding of their actions.

Within an organisation there may be a diverse range of simulation activities, from formal planned programmes to discrete sessions reflecting local incidents and events. In-situ training scenarios will need to be different from the ones used for planned sessions – in terms of learning aims, length and content. In-situ sessions are often run for any staff members who happen to be available, which may present a real challenge for the educator, who must subtly adjust the content and the scenario to fit the audience, maintaining credibility, authenticity and buy-in from the learners. This is a very different situation from a scenario run in a classroom setting for a known group. There will often be several faculty members involved in the scenario, and their roles should be discussed beforehand so that they are clear. Often one (or more) of the facilitators will be responsible for using the manikin, whilst a second facilitator runs the scenario and interacts with the learners. The debriefing stage may then require several faculty members.

The simulation scenario

The scenario itself has to be considered, as we will see in Chapters 2, 3 and 4. Firstly, it needs to allow the learner to put themselves in the situation (in other words, contextualise themselves); otherwise they will quickly build barriers and disengagement will occur. For instance, if I am running a session for a group of midwives and I introduce a scenario by saying 'Imagine that you are attending a patient in their 70s, who is having an acute coronary event', this will immediately create a barrier because a midwife cannot contextualise herself in that role. However, if I say 'Whilst escorting a post-delivery patient back to the ward, you are called over to assist a member of the ward staff who has just found one of their patients unresponsive', a midwife should be able to see herself in the situation and will therefore believe in the scenario.

The scenario has to be clinically realistic, as little things that are not correct can irritate learners and detract from their learning. Also, beware of drilling learners to respond to a standardised event to such an extent that they do not recognise a slightly different clinical presentation. For example, I have seen learners becoming so confident in responding to a particular type of manikin that they are completely thrown if that manikin is replaced by a real patient with pulses in slightly different locations.

The learners

The target learners are integral to the scenario, not only because the learning outcomes are aligned to their skills and needs but also because they need to be engaged by the scenario and 'buy in' to it. The majority of simulations run in practice will be seen as simulations and will never seem entirely real. If the learner does not 'play the game', the scenario will stall or even fail to start. This is partly why it is so important to make learners feel at ease by first introducing them to the equipment and scenario and setting clear ground rules. Clearly, expecting a group of student nurses to perform an emergency thoracotomy during a scenario would be unrealistic! In practice, we don't always know who will be available for a simulation so learning outcomes will need to be quite generic – for example, 'respond to the patient appropriately' or 'focus more on the team work and patient safety aspects'.

The limitations of simulation

Firstly, a manikin or actor is obviously not a real patient and cannot therefore give an entirely real experience. Secondly, it is not possible to recreate all the elements of typical working shifts. For instance, it is not normal practice to set up a scenario at 4am, when learners are tired. But of course in a real practice setting they may well be required to cope with such a situation in the early hours.

In addition, simulation equipment is expensive to buy and maintain and facilitators will be senior staff with extensive clinical and educational experience, and it will therefore be expensive to release them from clinical practice. Simulation is also a low throughput event. If larger groups are trained, the session will probably need to be repeated numerous times. As we have seen, simulation is not always the best learning tool. For instance, it is often easier, when teaching basic knowledge or theory, to use either a standard face-to-face teaching session (perhaps a lecture, seminar or working in small groups) or an e-learning presentation. This is why it is so important to see simulation in the context of blended learning activities.

Simulation and healthcare error

An awareness of error in healthcare is important, as errors can be identified and mitigated through simulation training. This can be accomplished by developing a team's awareness of the human factors that lead to errors and identifying situations in which errors are more likely to occur. Having identified errors in simulated events, we can try to prevent them recurring through learning and organisational change.

It is generally recognised that around 80% of errors are caused by the human element (Perrow 1984), either through human/human interaction or human/machine interaction. Communication is seen as a major contributor to these errors (Lee *et al.* 2012). It has been suggested in healthcare in the UK that up to 10% of patients admitted to hospital are at risk of a patient safety event (ASGBI 2010).

James Reason described the 'Swiss Cheese Model', which demonstrates how an error is propagated through a system (Reason 1997). According to this model, the error passes through the slices of 'cheese' with holes in them. The cheese slices represent systems and processes designed to prevent the error, and the holes represent active failures and latent conditions. This model demonstrates that most incidents and harm events are caused by a combination of multiple factors. One can often trace a chain of different errors and failures leading to the incident. 'Active errors' are those made on the front line, by those who are working with the patient (Varpio *et al.* 2008) and they may be mistakes, omissions or procedural violations (Reason 1997). In contrast, 'latent errors' are organisational factors within systems and processes that can play a role in harm events.

The rest of this book looks at the individual elements of the simulation process and also some important aspects of facilitating simulation in a specific area or location.

References

Alinier, G. (2010). Developing high-fidelity care simulation scenarios: A guide for educators and professionals. *Simulation Gaming*. **42** (9), 9–26.

Association of Surgeons of Great Britain and Ireland (ASGBI). (2010). *Patient safety: a consensus statement*. London: Association of Surgeons of Great Britain and Ireland.

Beaubien, J.M. & Baker, D.P. (2004). The use of simulation for training teamwork skills in health care: how low can you go?. *Quality and Safety in Health Care*. **13**, i51–i56.

Berragan, L. (2011). Simulation: An effective pedagogical approach for nursing? *Nurse Education Today*. **31**, 660–63.

Bland, A.J., Topping, A. & Wood, B. (2011) A concept analysis of simulation as a learning strategy in the education of undergraduate nursing students. *Nursing Education Today*, **31**, 664–70.

Bradley, P. & Postlethwaite, K. (2003). Simulation in clinical learning. *Medical Education*. **37** (1), 1–5.

Castanelli, D.J. (2009). The rise of simulation in technical skills teaching and the implications for training novices in anaesthesia. *Anaesthesia and Intensive Care*. **37**, 903–10.

Department of Health. (2011). *A framework for technology enhanced learning*. London: HMSO.

Dieckmann, P., Gaba, D. & Rall, M. (2007). Deepening the theoretical foundations of patient simulation in practice as social practice. *Simulation in Healthcare*. **2**, 183–93.

Donaldson, L. (2009). *Safer medical practice: machines, manikins and polo mints. 150 years of the annual report of the Chief Medical Officer: On the state of public health 2008*. London: HMSO.

Duvivier, R.J., van Dalen, J., Muijtjens, A.M., Moulaert, V., Van der Vleuten, C. & Scherpbier, A. (2011). The role of deliberate practice in the acquisition of clinical skills. *BMC Medical Education*. **11**, 101.

Gaba, D. (2004). The future vision of simulation in health care. *Quality and Safety in Health Care*. **13**, i2–i10.

Gough, S., Hellaby, M., Jones, N. & MacKinnon, R. (2012). A review of undergraduate interprofessional simulation-based education (IPSE). *Collegian*. **19** (3), 153–70.

Grant, D.J. & Marriage, S.C. (2012). Training using medical simulation. *Archives of Disease in Childhood*. **97**, 255–9.

Honey, P. & Mumford, A. (1982). *The Manual of Learning Styles*. London: P. Honey.

Hotchkiss, M., Biddle, C., & Fallacaro, M. (2002). Assessing the authenticity of the human simulation experience in anesthesiology. *AANA Journal*. **70**, 470–73.

Issenberg, S.B. (2006). The scope of simulation-based healthcare education. *Simulation in Healthcare*. **1**, 203–8.

Issenberg, S.B., McGaghie, W.C., Petrusa, E.R., Lee Gordon, D. & Scalese, R.J. (2005). Features and uses of high-fidelity medical simulations that lead to effective learning: A BEME systematic review. *Medical Teaching*. **27** (1), 10–28.

Issenberg, S.B. & Scalese, R.J. (2008). Simulation in health care education. *Perspectives in Biology and Medicine*. **51** (1), 31–46.

Knowles, M. (1980). *The Modern Practice of Adult Education*. Chicago, USA: Association Press/Follett.

Kolb, D.A. (1983). *Experiential Learning: Experience as the Source of Learning and Development*. New Jersey: Prentice Hall.

Lee, P., Allen, K. & Daly, M. (2012). A 'Communication and Patient Safety' training programme for all healthcare staff: can it make a difference? *British Medical Journal of Quality and Safety*. **21**, 84e–88. doi:10.1136/bmjqs-2011-000297.

McGaghie, W.C., Issenberg, S.B., Petrusa, E.R. & Scalese, R.J. (2010). A critical review of simulation-based medical education research: 2003–2009. *Medical Education*. **44**, 50–63.

MacKinnon R.J. (2011). Editorial: The rise of the collaborative inter-professional simulation education network? *Infant*. **7**, 6–8.

Perrow, C. (1999). *Normal Accidents: Living with High Risk Technologies*. Princeton, USA: Princeton University Press.

Reason, J.T. (1997). *Managing the Risks of Organizational Accidents*. Aldershot, UK: Ashgate Publishing Limited.

Tam, M. (2000). Constructivism, instructional design, and technology: Implications for transforming distance learning. *Educational Technology & Society*. **3** (2), 1436–4522.

Varpio, L., Hall, P., Lingard, L. & Schryer, C.F. (2008). Interprofessional communication and medical error: A reframing of research questions and approaches. *Academic Medicine*. **83** (10), S76–S81.

Weller, J.M., Nestel, D., Marshall, S.D., Brooks, P.M. & Conn, J.J. (2012). Simulation in clinical teaching and learning. *Medical Journal of Australia*. **196** (9), 1–5.

Yajamanyam, P.K., Sohi, D., King, S., Wilkey, O., Sinclair, H. (2012). Latent error detection during in-situ simulation training in a district general hospital. *Archives of Disease in Childhood*. **97** (1), A177.

Chapter 2

Scenario/programme development

Key points

- The starting point for scenario design is the learning outcomes
- Such outcomes should be learner-specific or generic team outcomes
- The scenario will also reflect local available resources, including faculty
- Scenarios should include expected actions and evidence base
- Scenarios should be peer-reviewed and validated

Developing a scenario

Writing a scenario presents many challenges, perhaps the main one being the writer's inability to predict all the potential actions of the learner. If a scenario is too prescriptive, it may fail because a learner never does that specific task. A degree of flexibility therefore needs to be built into the scenario (Alinier 2010). Scenarios should be based on sound theoretical knowledge (Cordeau 2012) and be evidence-based and peer-reviewed in order to be validated. Although it is often useful to base a scenario on a real case history to ensure credibility (Holland *et al.* 2008), it is important to realise that not all presentations are typical. It is also vital to protect the identity of the patient and ward area. It would be very awkward if it became clear that the case presented was from a specific area in which one of the learners worked, for example.

There are many reasons to run a simulation scenario, whether in practice or in a training area. You may just be running an isolated scenario, or a collection of different scenarios that reinforce and develop a range of topics in order to form a course or training programme. The planning process can be broken down for each scenario so that it does not become too onerous, although preparation even for a single simulation can take some time (Brewer 2011). It is also possible to use a relatively small number of scenarios and adapt them for different purposes, or change the patient history to present the candidates with what appears to be a completely different scenario. Having discovered that medical nursing staff members were reluctant to attend sessions that had surgical patients, I developed two separate courses with identical scenarios but different patient demographics. For instance, 'Bob' could either present with chest pain following admission for a hernia repair or with chest pain following admission with community-acquired pneumonia.

The starting point for scenario design should always be the desired learning outcomes. These learning outcomes may come from a number of different sources, depending on the nature of the learners. According to the actual time available, facilitators should have between one and four learning outcomes for each session (Alinier 2010). These learning outcomes may be cognitive, technical or behavioural (Halamek 2008), and this links to our earlier definition of simulation (see page 4). We also have to be aware that we may have different learning outcomes for different professional groups or even different grades within the same professional group. In a practice area, we may not even know who our candidates will be. In this situation, it is best to keep the learning outcomes as generic as possible. Facilitators can also consider looking at team learning outcomes, rather than specific ones for individual learners.

Consider a chest pain scenario. We may decide that we want the first person to recognise that the patient is unwell and respond appropriately (for example, a healthcare assistant should simply call for help, while a junior nurse might start patient observations and call for help). When running a scenario for a group of students/trainees, we also need to make sure that our learning outcomes are relevant to this particular group by mapping the scenario to their curriculum needs. If the learners are qualified staff, then this step is sometimes less clear. There are baselines that staff can be expected to meet, but there may be significant variations between staff members who work in acute and less acute areas, and between newly qualified and more experienced staff, as well as between those who enjoy emergency cases and those who don't. It may even be necessary to undertake a training needs analysis (Alinier 2010) or incorporate information from other organisational resources like performance development reviews.

Do not underestimate the importance of practising how to respond to what may be seen as 'a minor condition'. There is often a temptation to have 'Armageddon' scenarios that we feel will challenge the learners! However, this is sometimes based on a false assumption that all the learners are at the same high level of confidence and competence. In practice, this may not always be the case. A less dramatic scenario may be just as effective a learning tool for these learners, while the 'end of the world' scenario could leave them feeling overwhelmed and have a negative effect on their confidence. One can even run totally 'normal' scenarios, where there are no acute events at all. This can be particularly useful with trainee or newly qualified staff, to help them develop professional identity and confidence in a qualified role.

Deciding on learning outcomes

Sources of learning outcomes

- **If on an academic course – from the curriculum**
- **Personal development – related to knowledge, skills framework**
- **Generated by the learner – for instance, from a personal development review**
- **From governance issues – as a result of incidents or 'near misses'**
- **An institutional need – for example, to reinforce mandatory programmes or raise awareness of new equipment or procedures**
- **In response to national drivers, such as the Francis report (Francis 2013).**

It is important to view these learning outcomes holistically, within the context of the whole learning process. Ideally, the target skills, knowledge or behaviours will be reinforced elsewhere in the learner's experience and this will ensure that all the important key areas have been covered. For example, if the simulation is taking place in a practice area, it is important to have some collaboration with higher education institutions (HEIs). Likewise, in the HEIs there needs to be an overview of how simulation is incorporated into the entire curriculum and what simulation may be available in the practice environment, rather than viewing the session as a stand-alone element. This is known as curriculum integration (Issenberg *et al.* 2005).

In addition to the desired learning outcomes and the needs of particular learners, there are other considerations that influence scenario design and these are listed below.

Other factors to consider when designing a scenario

- **Reasons for choosing simulation**
- **Learners' level of training and scope of practice**
- **Skill mix of the learners**
- **Faculty availability**
- **Faculty skills**
- **Time available**
- **Equipment available**
- **Teaching area availability**

- **Validation of the scenario**
- **Links to previous scenarios/teaching sessions**
- **Method of assessing skills, knowledge and behaviour**
- **Evaluation of the learning event**
- **Expected outcomes**
- **Key debriefing points**
- **Number of learners who will require this session**
- **Evidence base for best practice.**

Other considerations when developing a simulation

As a starting point, it is useful to consider why you are considering running the simulation and whether it is actually the best modality to present these particular learning points. There needs to be a strategic overview, looking at the curriculum and continuing professional development process as a whole.

Faculty availability

The available faculty will also greatly influence how you run your scenario and also, to an extent, the choice of clinical scenario. The available faculty needs to be credible and needs expertise to develop the scenario. For example, they should be aware of potential dangers in training a group to respond to a false situation that will never occur, or drilling them only to recognise one presentation of a condition that may have a diverse range of symptoms.

The available faculty will often be limited. For instance, there may be times when you have to run sessions with only two faculty members – working the manikin, briefing and debriefing. Compare this to a session run in a simulation centre, where several facilitators and possibly several technicians may be present. As we have seen, there are many forms of simulation and they should all help to reinforce each other. It should also be remembered that the simulation centre has spent considerable time and money developing a realistic environment, which you can acquire for free by using a real clinical area! For more on the facilitator's role in running the scenario, see Chapter 4.

Identifying learners' needs

The other factor in constructing the scenario is the learners – firstly, the skills mix of the group and then their associated scope of practice. The professional level of the group will clearly affect the scenario construction. For instance, consider a patient with chest pain and the differing responses they would receive from five student nurses, compared to five qualified senior nurses, compared to a mixture of junior and senior nursing and medical staff. Often, with a junior uni-professional group, the scenario will rapidly grind to a halt as we reach the point where senior staff would normally intervene. This demonstrates one of the shortcomings of running uni-professional scenarios.

There is only one situation where I would expect learners to 'act' in another role or grade. This is when they are nearly qualified and we allow them to work in a qualified role. The simulation will then enable them to develop a greater understanding of their imminent scope of practice. However, it is always unacceptable to have a junior doctor playing a nurse, a nurse playing a physiotherapist, and so on. This serves only to reinforce negative stereotypes and leads to confusion on the part of the learners.

It is also important at this stage to consider how to assess whether the learners have achieved the expected level of competence at the end of the simulation. Evaluation of the learners is vital in order to measure the success of your scenario. It also gives you objective information on which to base your debriefing session. The assessment of the learners can obviously include whether they successfully used recognised national treatment guidelines or procedures. However, it may also be useful to look at team and leader responses and assess the human factor issues within the scenario. Various observational validated tools are available to guide an assessment of these skills and enable facilitators to make a more standardised, objective assessment. Using these tools, aligned to the learners' scope of practice, also increases the effectiveness of the assessment, debriefing and potential learning

Validating the scenario

There needs to be a validation process for the scenario. Typically, validation will consist of the scenario being peer-reviewed and linked to local or national standards. We may also involve learners, patient groups and organisational or national experts in developing the scenario. The simulation is then run as a pilot and further reviewed, following feedback from learners and faculty. You may additionally have access to a scenario bank, or scenarios from different institutions. However, these will have been designed for a specific situation and set of learning outcomes that may not match your own. It should always be remembered that a validated scenario was validated for a specific group or situation.

Evaluating the scenario

It is important that the evaluation phase of the scenario is included early on, and this includes evaluating the actions of the learners as well as evaluating the scenario. Evaluation helps to develop and improve any learning session. Feedback is typically obtained from the learners on how they enjoyed the session. However, this is very low-level feedback, as everyone usually enjoys simulation – especially if the patient recovers and we finish on time! Using validated tools to measure candidates' performance allows a higher level of evaluation.

Ultimately, we should be looking for even higher levels of evaluation that demonstrate changes in patient satisfaction and safety. This type of research and follow-up is usually too time-consuming to be practical but it is still very worthwhile in proving the importance of what you are doing as a facilitator. It is especially useful to revisit the learning outcomes at this stage, to see if any of these could be measured directly as an indicator. For instance, let's say that we have been asked to provide some simulation training in a ward area where there have been two recorded cases of delays in calling the cardiac arrest team. We could analyse the time taken to call for help before training (in-situ drill) and compare this to the time taken after training. For more information on evaluation, see Chapter 12.

A typical simulation scenario template

Let's say we have decided that our scenario is going to be about a patient who has an anaphylactic reaction. We can now develop the scenario, using a template to standardise the information. This template is helpful for scenario development, validation and facilitation, as all faculty members will become familiar with the way information is organised, under particular headings.

Scenario template

Title of the scenario

Overview of the scenario

Learning outcomes

Equipment/resources required

Assessment tools/process

Scenario learners' roles/professions

Background – setting the scene

Initial observations

Timeline of expected events

Key debriefing points

Review of evidence base/educational material

Documentation on validation process/authors

Background

The background contextualises the scenario, enabling the learners to see themselves in this created reality. It doesn't have to be a formal handover. We may just state that 'Bob was admitted yesterday to this (medical) ward with exacerbations of his COPD'. It is useful to give the patient a name in the scenario, as this allows all resources, such as X-rays, ECGs, drug charts and so on, to be clearly identified (Alinier 2010).

Next, we have to decide what has caused his anaphylaxis. The first thought will always be an antibiotic but perhaps he has been given an antibiotic because of a suspected chest infection? This may be appropriate for a group of junior learners but in my opinion antibiotics is one of those 'red flag' words that just screams 'anaphylactic scenario'. (In the same way, the words 'post-operative patient' immediately make learners think of a 'post-operative bleed'.) I have run an anaphylaxis training session and the first scenario was a *non-anaphylaxis* patient purely and simply because the candidates expected it to be anaphylaxis, as it was an anaphylaxis session. In this way, I sowed doubt in their minds and made them think about the actual diagnosis. The second scenario was a food-mediated reaction with a patient who developed a rash but did not immediately require adrenaline. The third was full-blown anaphylaxis with stridor. This allowed me to show a range of triggers and presentations and broaden the experience of the learners, allowing for a situation that occurs rarely in practice.

Initial observations

We now need to decide on our baseline patient observations – the first set of observations that we reveal. Remember, often the first observations required will be the ones when the patient deteriorates, unless the patient is monitored before. This is helpful because it can minimise programming or manual changes, and the manikin can be initially set ready for the deterioration.

Timeline of expected events

At this point, we can list our expected actions (either team or individual), again linking them to our learners' scope of practice. We also need to consider what we will do if the learners don't carry out the expected actions. It is not possible to think of every eventuality but there will be some obvious ones, such as not recognising the condition or not treating it appropriately. It has been suggested that the scenario should be shown as a flow diagram with multiple paths (Alinier 2010). Important steps need to be identified and faculty made aware of the learning outcomes so that deviation from the scenario can be recognised and a response can be prepared. This will be discussed further in Chapter 4.

The next consideration is how quickly these patient observations change. As a rule, they need to alter slowly enough to give time for the learners to respond and act. If they change too quickly, we risk ending up with the patient so acutely unwell that we have little room to make them worse. For instance, a patient with an oxygen saturation of 78% who is still not on oxygen will be heading for a hypoxic arrest and there will be nothing the learners can do.

Review of evidence base

It is useful to attach the underpinning clinical evidence basis for treatment to the scenario. This allows novice facilitators to expand their knowledge in the scenario field and confirms which documents expected actions are based on. It also provides a list of potential resources for learners before or after the scenario, and helps to demonstrate that the scenario and expected outcomes are up to date and reflect current practice.

Key debriefing points

Our scenario document framework (see Scenario Template, page 22) will also have some key debriefing points, which are often based on the learning outcomes. However, if we have several scenarios, there may be some key outcomes that are common to several of them. For instance, the scenarios may all aim to encourage effective communication as a learning outcome. It maybe that in the first scenario a key debriefing point would focus on why effective communication is important, whilst a later scenario focuses on how this may be achieved. The key debriefing points are supplemented by others which are generated by the students' activity.

Documentation on validation process

The next stage will involve a group of subject experts reading through the scenario and agreeing that it is valid. This group of experts can be sourced locally. For example, it could be a group of consultant obstetricians and senior midwives reviewing an obstetric scenario. It should also include experts in the use of simulation. Finally, it is often useful to trial the scenario with a combined group of facilitators and learners, to iron out any issues and problems that may have not been anticipated earlier (Alinier 2010).

After the scenario has been developed

The scenario is now complete. It has been validated in terms of the clinical course and expected actions, and it is up to date and evidence-based. Despite the use of a robust planning process, the scenario will often develop and evolve over time (Holland *et al.* 2008) and require further modification. It will also be necessary to review the content regularly, to ensure that there have been no alterations in practice or guidelines.

The modality of simulation being used to run the scenario will dictate the next step. For example, it may now be necessary to program the manikin to respond in an appropriate way. Alternatively, we may decide to run the scenario without programming in real time, or have a paper crib sheet and interject with patient observations. We may need to write a briefing sheet for a standardised patient or engage with someone who has the knowledge to develop a virtual scenario.

Having developed and validated a scenario based on our learners' scope of practice with clearly identified learning outcomes, we have piloted this to produce a scenario which should be fit for practice. The next chapter will explore how we introduce this scenario to our learners.

References

Alinier, G. (2010). Developing high-fidelity care simulation scenarios: A guide for educators and professionals. *Simulation Gaming*. **42** (9), 9–26.

Brewer, E.P. (2011). Successful techniques for using human patient simulation in nursing education. *Journal of Nursing Scholarship*. **43** (3), 311–17.

Cordeau, M.A. (2012). Linking the transition, a substantive theory of high-stakes clinical simulation. *Advances in Nursing Science*. **35** (3), E90–E102.

Francis, R. (2013). *Report of the Mid Staffordshire NHS Foundation Trust Public Inquiry*. London: HMSO.

Halamek, L. (2008). The simulated delivery-room environment as the future modality for acquiring and maintaining skills in fetal and neonatal resuscitation. *Seminal Fetal Neonatal Medicine*. **13**, 448–53.

Holland, C., Sadler, C. & Nunn, A. (2008). *Scenario Design: Theory to Delivery in Manual of Simulation in Healthcare*. Oxford: Oxford University Press.

Issenberg, S.B., McGaghie, W.C., Petrusa, E.R., Lee Gordon, D. & Scalese, R.J. (2005). Features and uses of high-fidelity medical simulations that lead to effective learning: A BEME systematic review. *Medical Teaching*. **27** (1), 10–28.

Chapter 3

Introducing the scenario

Key points

During the introduction, we need to:

- Establish a safe learning environment
- Establish what we are expecting learners to do
- Familiarise learners with the manikin
- Brief the learners

The scenario has been planned, mapped, piloted and validated, and the facilitators have a thorough understanding of the needs of the learners, and the learning outcomes. With all this in place, we can now prepare to run the scenario by welcoming and briefing the students.

The purpose of the briefing stage

The briefing stage is not often described in depth in articles (Husebø *et al.* 2012).

Essentially, it is used to foster a safe learning environment, establish what is expected in the session, set ground rules for behaviour, familiarise the learners with the simulation area and equipment and answer any questions. Husebø *et al.* suggest that the briefing stage is often taken for granted even though it offers a vital opportunity to assess whether learners have an understanding of the instructions, and to clarify them if necessary. They also stress the importance of clarifying the specific elements that will be attempted, to avoid ambiguity and confusion (*ibid.*).

Establishing a safe learning environment

Establishing a safe learning environment and learning climate is really important. When the facilitator explains why the session is being run, some of the candidates will worry that there is an element of summative assessment. They may even be concerned about why they have been selected to do the session and also about what will happen if they 'fail'. In order to allay such fears, the learning event needs to be set in the context of developing skills and using formative assessment with feedback. Simulation is often a new experience for learners (Jeffries 2005). Because of the lack of clarity about the use of the term, even those who think they have undertaken simulation before may actually have done something quite different.

Reassure the learners that you appreciate that they have previous experience and knowledge and that you welcome them in sharing and reflecting on relevant previous experiences. It is useful to explain that the scenarios are designed to be a challenge and that learners are allowed to make mistakes in this controlled area. These will not result in patient harm and can be discussed openly later.

At this stage, it is important to instill the idea of you being a facilitator (rather than a lecturer or hierarchical management figure). Confidentiality must also be discussed, for a number of reasons. Firstly, it is not desirable to have learners openly discussing with colleagues how a particular person performed. In addition, discussing the scenarios with peers who may attend the session in the future will detract from their learning experience.

There is a slight ethical dilemma here. Should you tell the learners that their responses will be kept explicitly confidential – in other words, 'what happens in the scenario stays in the scenario'? This may indeed be beneficial in helping to reassure the learners. However, there are very rare occasions when an individual's behaviour, skills or knowledge give such cause for concern that you may need to consider taking further action. This can be an especially pressing issue when running in-situ sessions with qualified staff – because these staff will return directly to clinical practice following the session. There needs to be some planned response to the learner in difficulty, and steps must be agreed to minimise any potential patient risk. Because of this, I do not explicitly state that the faculty will not discuss people's actions with others – and, interestingly, I have never had a candidate question me on this. At this point, it may also be necessary to gain learners' consent to video the session. Such consent should be in writing and must include precise explanation of what the videos will be used for.

Establishing what learners are expected to do

Your expectations of learners will be affected by various elements of the scenario. Often, it is sufficient to state that you expect them to work within their scope of practice, to call for help when they would normally do so, and to treat the patient as a real patient. It is also worth explaining the limitations of the manikin with a general statement such as 'At the end of this introduction I will show you exactly what the manikin can and cannot do. However, if there is anything you would normally do to a patient, we would expect you to do this to the manikin'. This is also the point to clarify what you expect them to do (and not do) so they understand what is involved.

The structure of the session should be explained, especially how the scenario and debriefing session will be run, in order to overcome learners' fear of the unknown. At this point, it is useful to set the ground rules regarding behaviour and open communication, whereby team members review each other's performance without being judgemental (Arafeh *et al.* 2010). I often explain that I will not have everyone start the scenario together, and emphasise again that the learners need to act within their scope of practice. For a novice group, I also say that the scenario will run at a slower pace and we can discuss things or even pause along the way. I have found that this works well in practice. More advanced learners may find interruptions a distraction but a careful facilitator can add questions during the scenario, as a team member might raise a particular concern during the simulation.

You also need to tell the learners how you are going to run the scenario. I normally explain that I will present them with the scenario and then nominate who responds. Everyone will have a go. This means that you can put weaker and stronger learners in pairs, and let them work collaboratively to solve problems together (Jeffries 2005). I also explain the debriefing process that we will use and tell the learners that we can answer any questions at this stage.

In effect, what you are doing is confirming that the session is aligned to adult learning theory – though some of these concepts are somewhat manipulated. For example, the learners may appear to be leading the scenario, while in fact the facilitator is steering it. You may also decide to disclose some or all of the learning aims and outcomes for the scenario, particularly if they are generic. For instance, saying 'In this scenario we will look at developing our team working and leadership skills' may be more useful than simply establishing that one of the outcomes is to diagnose anaphylaxis in a patient.

Familiarising learners with the manikin

This may be the first time that these learners have been involved in a simulation and they may have various preconceptions, worries and fears. They may be worried about the simulation process in general, puzzled about the rationale for using simulation and apprehensive about using the equipment. Remember that they may never have seen a manikin more advanced than the ones commonly used for resuscitation. Because of this, they will not understand how you want them to interact with the manikin or standardised patient.

There are a couple of ways to familiarise the learners with the manikin. One way is to physically give the learners 'a tour'. This would include what we can and can't do with a manikin. For instance, if your manikin set-up will not display oxygen saturation, you need to tell them how they find out what the oxygen saturation is. I usually run through a very basic demonstration – typically I use the standard ABCDE (Airway, Breathing, Circulation, Disability, Exposure) examination and ask them to talk me through what to do. This has several purposes. Firstly, it standardises the learner's approach to using the ABCDE examination. Secondly, it introduces the roles of the multi-professional team. Thirdly, it allows me to show them what the manikin can do, and its limitations, and how I can give the learners any additional information they may require. It also shows that the facilitator is willing to step up in front of the learners and makes it more likely that the learners will volunteer in the actual scenario.

Briefing the learners

Finally, you need to give the learners the relevant background information on the patient. This may be done in the form of a formal brief or perhaps more often as part of a shift handover, from one member of staff to another. This will provide an opportunity to summarise pertinent background information and also an opportunity for the learners to ask questions. There may be occasions when only minimal information is given, and the team will be expected to find out the information as they go, as may happen in an emergency situation. The next chapter looks at how we facilitate the simulation session.

References

Arafeh, J.M.R., Snyder Hansen, S. & Nichols, A. (2010). Debriefing in simulated-based learning: Facilitating a reflective discussion. *Journal of Perinatal and Neonatal Nursing*. **24** (4), 302–309.

Jeffries, P.R. (2005). A framework for designing, implementing, and evaluating simulations used as teaching strategies in nursing. *Nursing Education Perspectives*. **26** (2), 96–103.

Husebø, S.E., Friberg, F., Søreide, E. & Rystedt, H. (2012). Instructional problems in briefings: How to prepare nursing students for simulation-based cardiopulmonary resuscitation training. *Clinical Simulation in Nursing*. **8** (7), e307–e318. doi:10.1016/j.ecns.2010.12.002.

Chapter 4

Running the scenario

Key points

- The availability of faculty will determine how you run the session
- The facilitator needs to be familiar with the scenario
- Cueing can be performed in a variety of covert and overt ways
- Cueing is subjective and a learnt skill but can be incorporated into the scenario
- Within the scenario, the facilitator will need to compensate for the ways in which the manikin and the equipment used differ from real life

You have now introduced the session and you are ready to run the scenario. The way you actually run the scenario will depend on the equipment you have available, the available faculty and support staff and your chosen location.

Within the hospital environment, experienced facilitators are a scarce resource. The term 'facilitator' implies that the person running the scenario also participates in it, guiding and steering it to meet the aims of the session. This can be a very light-handed approach, using simple questions and statements or even modifying the responses of the manikin. So where should the facilitator be during the session? They can be overtly in the room as a member of the faculty, covertly in the room in the guise of another candidate, or somewhere between the two – perhaps as 'an extra' in the scenario, undertaking a role as a relative, or as a more junior staff member who would not be expected to be drawn into the action of the case. The seniority and skill mix of the group will help to dictate the exact role of the facilitator, with more experienced teams requiring less input.

What does the facilitator do during the scenario?

- **Provides information**
- **Keeps the scenario moving**
- **Keeps the scenario on track by questioning, hinting or giving cues**
- **Deals with equipment issues**
- **Operates equipment for the learners**
- **Knows how to operate extraneous equipment (e.g. monitors and infusion pumps)**
- **Makes up for lack of manikin/simulation reality**
- **Provides feedback to manikin operator**
- **Provides feedback for faculty debriefing (or carries out debriefing)**
- **Monitors and intervenes in any observed risk-taking**
- **May increase psychological fidelity (e.g. by acting as parent of patient).**

When and how to cue

Clearly, the facilitator has to have a thorough knowledge of the scenario, as one of the most important tasks will be that of giving cues or prompts in order to keep it on track. Jeffries suggests that there is often a lack of clarity around how and when cues are delivered (Jeffries 2005). There are various ways to give cues but the first consideration is *when* to cue – if the session starts to diverge from the planned scenario. This decision will partly depend on how big a divergence it is, and whether it will still allow the learning objectives to be obtained. If not, either the scenario should be stopped immediately and there should be a discussion about where it's going, or the facilitator should re-start the session or steer the learners back on course by using verbal or non-verbal prompts or manipulating manikin parameters.

Within the scenario, there will be certain documented actions that need to occur so that the scenario stays on track and learning outcomes are met. These will be the main items that will need to be cued.

Consider the simple scenario of treating an asthmatic patient. One of the expected outcomes will be the application of high-flow oxygen to the patient. However, after a predefined point in a particular session, it becomes obvious that the candidates are not considering oxygen therapy.

The facilitator has a number of options. The first is to do nothing – and use this as a point for debriefing afterwards, even though this omission could constitute a serious deviation from the scenario. What if it was a more concerning deviation or drug error, which would stop the scenario entirely? There are different schools of thought. One would say 'Let them run with it. They will learn from the mistake and it will be unlikely to occur again'. Personally, in this situation I would probably intervene, once it was clear that the omission or error was going to occur but before they actually did it.

Secondly, you could offer a verbal prompt such as 'The patient looks very blue'. This should make them reflect on what is going on and what they have forgotten! In such situations, you may feel you are dragging the learners through the scenario, rather than steering them. However, giving this type of cue still produces a more positive outcome than letting the candidates fail and doing nothing.

Finally, you could change a parameter on the patient monitor. In this case, the patient/manikin will continue to desaturate and you will hope that one of the learners notices.

Often, a facilitator will need to escalate the overtness of the cue – starting with the subtle and becoming less subtle. However, there will come a point where the facilitator has to decide whether to physically instruct the learners to perform a task (to enable the scenario to continue) or to let the scenario continue without it. Either option can be discussed and investigated during the debriefing. A lot of the decisions about when to cue or not come from previous experience with that particular scenario, knowledge of the norms of the group and of course the scenario itself.

Finally, the facilitator always has to be ready for the sudden bizarre question or request that could lead the scenario off on a tangent. Most of the time these requests can be met with a stock answer such as 'That is not available on this ward/area' or 'We have asked for it/It is on the way.'

Dealing with death

A lot of centres decide beforehand that 'the patient' will not die during the scenario, except when this is written in as part of the learning outcomes. It is therefore necessary for the facilitator to stop any potentially fatal action occurring, such as a junior doctor giving an IV bolus of 30mg morphine for pain relief. The main reason not to include death is that the candidates may feel grief, guilt, blame and anger, which will disrupt the learning process. We will also have to reset the scenario and manikin. Depending on the type of manikin and programming method, this may take some time.

Deciding who goes first

The learning experience should be a pleasurable one. Candidates may be nervous and apprehensive, so you must be aware that your engagement and interactions with them will be remembered. Also, if you are not careful, certain comments can backfire. For example, a seemingly innocent joke at a candidate's expense can lead to the candidates joining ranks against you as the facilitator.

In a multi-professional group, you will have already decided which professional groups will attend first, and this will limit your choice of candidates. Care must be taken when selecting which candidates to go in first. I always keep an eye on the candidates initially, observing their body language and level of confidence. If you have a couple of apparently weaker, nervous junior staff, consider sending them in together so that they can support each other and act as they would in a real ward situation. Sending in individuals on their own would make it seem more like a test. It's also a good idea to mix teams up, rather than having two separate teams that alternate scenarios. Again, this reflects the haphazard nature of real healthcare action teams.

Problems that may be encountered during a scenario

What can go wrong during the scenario?

- **There may be a lack of fidelity (for example, the manikin or environment could significantly differ from reality)**
- **A candidate may be unfamiliar with an item of equipment**
- **A candidate may not be familiar with the manikin (despite introductory explanation)**
- **There may be an argumentative candidate in the group**
- **A confrontation could take place between two candidates**
- **A candidate may be upset**
- **A candidate may be over-dominant and try to 'take over' the session**
- **Candidate(s) may not want to participate in the session**
- **There could be a technical failure**
- **A candidate may carry out an unexpected action**
- **A candidate may do something that could be hazardous to other learners or themselves.**

Compensating for lack of manikin fidelity

As the manikin is not a real person, there are areas that it cannot mimic or replicate so we need to find other ways of providing this information for the learners. Consider an anaphylaxis scenario. A basic manikin will not be able to develop a rash, and yet 80% of patients who develop anaphylaxis will. Clearly, we need to make the candidates aware that they should look for a rash. We could:

- prepare the manikin with a rash, drawn on the skin
- inform the learners that the patient looks 'very flushed'
- develop some technology to allow a rash to appear (Hellaby 2011).

The decision on which path is taken will depend on such factors as the skill of the facilitator, the time allowed between scenarios, and how often the scenario is run. There is no single correct solution but this type of issue will certainly affect the realism of the session. It will also be relatively easy to anticipate during the planning stage so some preparation can be made for it.

Preparing for the debrief

Another aspect we need to think about is how we record information for the debrief. We will have already considered what details we are going to assess and how we are going to do this. We now need to work through the scenario, paying attention to timing. It is easy to let the scenario run on and then find that there is too little time left for debriefing. Having reached the concluding stage, the facilitator needs to announce that the scenario is finished and prepare for the debriefing, which is discussed in the next chapter.

References

Jeffries, P.R. (2005). A framework for designing, implementing, and evaluating simulations used as teaching strategies in nursing. *Nursing Education Perspectives*. **26** (2), 96–103.

Hellaby, M.D. (2011). Anaphylaxis simulation session: Seeing is believing. *Simulation in Healthcare*. **6** (3), 180–83

Chapter 5

Debriefing

Key points

- Debriefing is a critical part of the simulation process
- Debriefing is the time when we turn actions into learning and put change into practice
- The emotional climate of the debriefing needs to be established
- The facilitator takes on the role of co-learner to explore actions using good judgement and advocacy with enquiry
- Debriefing uses a reflective process
- Debriefing expertise is developed over time and requires faculty development

Debriefing within the simulated learning event is recognised as vital (Issenberg *et al.* 2005, Arafeh *et al.* 2010, McGaghie *et al.* 2010) in order to maximise learning (Fanning & Gaba 2007). Debriefing has various aims but the most important is to facilitate an active discussion of events to synergise, strengthen and transfer learning from the experience (Warrick *et al.* 1979). Ruth Fanning and David Gaba (2007) described debriefing as a 'facilitated or guided reflection in the cycle of experiential learning'. It is the time when we can turn actions (or lack of actions) into learning. The ultimate goal is translational learning, where reflection leads not just to changes in knowledge, skills and/or behaviour in the subsequent simulation but also to changes in clinical practice.

However, it is fair to say that the importance of the debrief is often unacknowledged and it can frequently be an afterthought, with only a few moments left at the end of a session to summarise the main learning outcomes (Arafeh *et al.* 2010). When performed well, debriefing can be effective, constructive and enjoyable. However, if performed badly it has the potential to confuse learners, reduce their confidence (*ibid.*) and tarnish the reputation of simulation in general. Debriefing is often the aspect that simulation faculty feel least confident with. Many facilitators are senior clinicians and practitioners, who understand and feel comfortable with running the scenarios but may be less familiar and comfortable with the theoretical approaches required in debriefing.

Debriefing has been described as an art rather than a skill (Fanning & Gaba 2007). It is not something that one can pick up by reading a book – it requires time, effort and reflection to master. Good debriefers are keen to receive feedback from learners and peers and always reflect on each session. This chapter can only offer an introduction to the subject of debriefing, which in truth requires a book in its own right.

Notice that we are discussing debriefing, as opposed to feedback. Feedback tends to suggest a statement of events and performance, whereas debriefing is much more of a two-way interactive and reflective process.

The purpose of debriefing

The aims of debriefing

- **To resolve conflicts**
- **To answer questions on performance from learners**

- **To answer other questions**
- **To confirm that learning outcomes have been recognised and met**
- **To enable and guide a reflective experience**
- **To help establish an action plan for future situations**
- **To aim for translational learning (a change in clinical practice).**

Debriefing serves all these purposes, some of which are required to optimise the learning climate. Wickers (2010) describes the atmosphere of security that the facilitator has to create in order to decrease learners' anxiety. We need to explain the debriefing process, if we have not already done this, and again reinforce that this is a safe place for the students to express their thoughts and feelings. As part of this, we will also often discuss ground rules for the learners (Arafeh *et al.* 2010), emphasising that this is a positive learning event.

There may have been conflict during the scenario, or the learners may be so 'caught up' in the action that there needs to be a formal end to the scenario and a chance to de-escalate emotions. This is often initiated with the facilitator stating that the scenario has ended. Physically moving the learners from the simulation area to a debriefing area also helps to emphasise the transition, as does the layout of the area. An area set up with chairs in a circle reinforces the fact that we are all equal in the debriefing session. Questions need to be answered. Often there is a fixation on specific clinical actions and decisions. There may also be an acknowledgement that certain steps were omitted. It is important to resolve all these issues.

The role of the facilitator in debriefing

The facilitator can significantly influence the climate of the debriefing session. It is not just a question of what the facilitator does; it is the whole atmosphere that is developed through the facilitator's demeanour (Neill & Wotton 2011). As the learners need to be actively involved in the discussion, the facilitator's role is ideally that of a co-learner, who is going to explore the events that have occurred so that the group can better understand them. This is quite different from the role of lecturer or instructor, which has connotations of an authority gradient.

In accordance with this approach, we need to get away from the idea that the facilitator is correct (always) and the learner is incorrect (often). Instead, we need to develop a debriefing 'with good judgement' (Rudolph *et al.* 2007). We need to examine the actions, or lack of actions, that occurred and try to understand the reasons for them. Jenny Rudolph and her colleagues describe this as a different way of talking, by combining advocacy with inquiry (*ibid.*). In their article, they describe debriefings as being judgemental, non-judgemental or run with good judgement. The judgemental debriefing does not encourage learning, serves only to reinforce the instructor's position of power and results in defensiveness on the part of the learner. In the non-judgemental debrief, the facilitator often ends up hiding the underlying message that there is something the learner should have done. The non-judgemental debrief gives the learner confusing signals. The facilitator feels they cannot raise concerns, discuss poor performance or be confrontational (Rudolph *et al.* 2006). In contrast, it has been suggested that debriefing with good judgement, using advocacy with enquiry, allows us to mutually explore what happened in order to further the understanding of all (Rudolph *et al.* 2007).

The central tenet of debriefing with good judgement is to explore the learners' thought process that leads to their actions, from their viewpoint (Arafeh *et al.* 2010). These viewpoints, or frames, depend on many variables, assumptions and misconceptions, as well as previous knowledge and experience. Exploring all these factors utilises the experience and knowledge of the group, including that of the facilitator (co-learner), which can lead to the creation of new frames. The knowledge of the facilitator is thus used collectively, together with the insights of the other learners (Rudolph *et al.* 2007).

Consider a simulation situation in which you have noticed that a learner did not apply oxygen to a hypoxic patient. Let's look at the different stances you could adopt in the debriefing session:

- **Judgemental:** 'Why did you not put oxygen on?'
- **Non-judgemental:** 'Could you have put oxygen on?'
- **Good judgement:** 'I was concerned that you didn't give supplemental oxygen to the patient. I realise there were a lot of priorities in managing the case (advocacy) but I'm curious about how you saw them? (inquiry)'

In this instance, using advocacy with inquiry enables the facilitator to explore the thought process behind their actions. This can also give the facilitator a useful opportunity to avoid possible embarrassment. It is always rather awkward to tackle an apparently sub-standard learner and start critiquing their behaviour, only to discover that, once they have justified their thought process, their actions appear in a different light or that you simply missed them performing a specific action.

The structure of the debrief

Historically, other models have been used to structure the medical education debrief, such as the Feedback sandwich and Pendleton's Rules (Bullock *et al.* 2008).

Table 5.1: **Previous debriefing models**

	Feedback (Positive) Sandwich	**Pendleton's Rules**
Description	• Tell them what went well in first attempt • Tell them where they could improve • Tell them about another aspect that went well	• Ask them what went well • Tell them what you think they did well • Ask them what they would like to improve • Tell them what you think they should do differently
Potential pitfalls	• Instructor led, maintains learner/instructor divide • Emphasises positive events • Can lose credibility of learners	• Learners often don't feel they did anything well • They may not be aware of what they could do to improve

Adapted from Bullock *et al.* 2008.

Whilst potentially providing the novice faculty member with a clear guide, these models are often too rigid and may even be misleading. Think of the learner who has acted with very little insight throughout the simulation, and has not adhered to proven practice or standards. In this case, it would be difficult to use the sandwich method (good feedback/improvement feedback/good feedback) for several reasons. Firstly, the learner may lose sight of the fact that they have performed sub-optimally because there was only one 'bad' thing and two 'good'. Secondly, the facilitator may lose credibility with the other learners, who will recognise that their peer's actions leave room for improvement.

There are numerous models for facilitating a debriefing session, and these will commonly have reflective practice and experiential learning at their core (Fanning & Gaba 2007). There tend to be three discrete phases during the debrief (Arafeh *et al.* 2010). These three phases have been given many different names but they are all based on the idea of synergising, strengthening and transferring learning (Warrick *et al.* 1979). These steps can be seen as part of a reflective process. Indeed it has been suggested that a debriefing can foster reflective practice (Dreifuerst 2009), increasing novice reflectors' experience with the reflective process and enabling them to use the process in clinical practice, which may help them develop clinical judgement (Mayville 2011). It is therefore sensible for the facilitator to use a reflective process that is recognised by the learners and guide them through the process. This reflective process may be repeated a number of times for individual elements of enquiry.

Potential issues during the debriefing

There are various potential problems and conflicts that may be encountered during the debriefing process. These include:

- Disengagement
- Argumentative candidate/s
- Failure by candidate/s to accept that their behaviour/actions caused specific issues
- Fixation on poor performance
- Defensiveness against potential criticism
- Conflict with other learners
- Lack of reflective engagement.

You will notice that this list is similar to the list of problems that can arise while running the scenario.

Defensiveness against perceived criticism is a natural response and needs to be handled sensitively. Learners commonly make statements such as 'I wouldn't do that to a real patient.' I often agree that the manikin isn't real and we recognise that, but when we reflect on practice it may turn out that many of the team have seen similar events. Again, this encourages learners to reflect on their actions.

One way that perceived perceptions can be addressed is to physically demonstrate the issue to the learner. This may be by simply asking a fellow team member how they felt when a particular situation occurred – although this does require a peer to speak up to a colleague or senior and it can therefore be a risky strategy with certain team dynamics.

Video-assisted feedback is generally more effective, though the cost, technical skills required and ethical issues involved may preclude it being used on every occasion and in every setting. In its simplest form, a real-time video is taken of the session and this is replayed – stopping, rewinding and replaying to facilitate the debrief. As the majority of the playback will not be needed, it requires some skill to locate the relevant points/areas and this may cause a distraction. A further refinement would be to utilise video capture software, which can allow the user to identify and tag key events and label these for ease of retrieval during the debriefing. This allows instant feedback of pertinent points and also allows video to be captured as part of a more structured debriefing process. However, video does present some issues in itself. For example, the idea of being filmed can be very off putting for the participants. We also need to get consent to record any images and we will need to explicitly state what we will be doing with the recordings. The majority of centres will delete the recordings following the session. If they are being kept you will need to state why and who they will be shown to. They will also need to be stored securely.

Observational metrics, whether non-technical or technical skill score sheets, can be used to rate an individual's behaviour and provide objective data, which may be used in the debrief. Observational metrics are also available for team (as well as individual) behaviour and even for roles within the team. Using metrics has the advantage of turning a subjective impression into a more objective assessment, and sometimes exemplars of activity can be used to further explain individual points.

Clearly, it will not be possible to debrief the entire scenario, as schedules and faculty/learner attention will not allow the session to continue for too long. The facilitator will therefore need to target the debrief to ensure that it covers key issues, questions from the learners and also any important issues that may have arisen during the session. The facilitator may want to steer the debrief to cover a specific area – perhaps aligned to key debriefing points – but it is important that other important events are not ignored. Remember that it is possible to engineer the scenario so that the key debriefing points become so fundamental that they need to be discussed anyway. For instance, running a scenario in which a key debriefing point is communication, in a place where there is a high ambient noise level, will mean that it needs to be discussed anyway. It is quite common to have decided on two or three items you as the facilitator wish to cover and have the learners bring these up before you do.

As already stated, debriefing is not a skill that can be learnt from a book. It requires practice, trial and error, and reflection. Consider how you would manage the following situations that commonly arise during debriefing.

The learner refuses to acknowledge any observed deficiencies

If video feedback is available, this will be very useful to help reinforce what you are suggesting. It may also help increase the learner's awareness of their need to make improvements if they can engage with other group members – though care needs to be taken, as team dynamics, working relationships and hierarchies may make it difficult for other faculty members or learners to give a truthful answer about this particular learner's performance. There are some candidates with very poor self-awareness and your management of the situation may be restricted by the length of the session. However, there is often a chance to return to the subject later in the course – ideally in a non-confrontational way that gives the person food for thought and encourages them to reflect.

The really good team/scenario

Do not be frightened to tell the individuals and team that they were very good, and do not feel that you have to force a debrief or feedback process. It is still possible to reflect on the learning outcomes, even if they have accomplished them all.

Conflict in the group

Scenarios are often designed to be challenging and may therefore become emotionally charged. There is also the added pressure of 'performing' in front of seniors and peers, and this may mean that conflict or dispute occasionally occur. The first thing that needs to be done is to recognise that the session is over by saying, for example, 'OK, that was obviously quite a challenging scenario so let's just catch our breath before we have a chat about it.'

One of the main purposes of the debrief is to resolve any outstanding issues. Allowing the conflict to remain unresolved would leave 'open wounds' and distract the learners. Obviously, it needs to be dealt with sensitively. It may be that one of the parties is unaware of the issue, in which case a simple question may suffice, such as 'I heard you ask twice if you should defibrillate the patient and didn't get a response. I was wondering how this made you feel?' If the conflict is obvious to both parties, it may be sufficient to carefully examine the situation that occurred and look at other non-confrontational strategies that could have been used. The aim is to provide some understanding of what has happened and how it has been interpreted. There may also be times when a line simply has to be drawn under the situation so as not to stall the course. If necessary, the discussion can be continued at another time with those involved.

A learner gets upset

If this occurs, the distressed learner should be spoken to separately from the group to ascertain the cause of the upset. If it is something that can be easily resolved, then the learner can be reintroduced. There will also be times where the clinical scenario may be too similar to a recent difficult case or a even family event. Often, with some discussion and clarity over the issue, they can rejoin the group, once they have recovered their composure. I can only recollect one occasion when I 'lost' a learner for good. This person had a phobia about manikins. The learner was doing well right up to the point when the manikin groaned at them – the next thing I saw was the doors swinging shut!

The evolving process of debriefing

As stated earlier, the debriefing process evolves with experience and peer review, and observation by an experienced debriefer can be useful to gain further insight. There are also metrics that can be used to assess the debriefing process such as the Debriefing Assessment for Simulation in Healthcare (DASH) (Simon *et al.* 2009). Because debriefing is so important, it should be assessed more often. Some centres are installing cameras in their debriefing areas so that faculty can review their performance, performance can be rated and faculty performance improved. Such faculty development is to be commended. There is a need for further research into optimum debriefing strategies and techniques, and an even greater need to explicitly describe the debriefing process and demonstrate its ability to affect patient outcomes (Raemer *et al.* 2011).

References

Arafeh, J.M.R., Snyder Hansen, S. & Nichols, A. (2010). Debriefing in simulated-based learning facilitating a reflective discussion. *Journal of Perinatal and Neonatal Nursing.* **24** (4), 302–9.

Bullock, I., Davis, M., Lockey, A. & Mackway-Jones, K. (2008). *Pocket Guide to Teaching for Medical Instructors.* (2nd ed.) London: Blackwell Publishing.

Dreifuerst, K.T. (2009). The essentials of debriefing in simulation learning: a concept analysis. *Nursing Education Perspectives.* **30** (2), 109–14.

Fanning, R.M. & Gaba, D.M. (2007). The role of debriefing in simulation-based learning. *Simulation in Healthcare.* **2**,115–25.

Issenberg, S.B., McGaghie, W.C., Petrusa, E.R., Gordon, D.L. & Scalese, R.J. (2005). Features and uses of high-fidelity medical simulations that lead to effective learning: a BEME systematic review. *Medical Teacher,* **27** (1), 10–28.

Mayville, M.L. (2011). Debriefing: The essential step in simulation. *Newborn and Infant Nursing Reviews.* **11** (1). 35–9.

McGaghie, W.C., Issenberg, S.B., Petrusa, E.R. & Scalese, R.J. (2010). A critical review of simulation-based medical education research: 2003–2009. *Medical Education.* **44**, 50–63. doi:10.1111/j.1365-2923.2009.03547.x

Neill, M.A. & Wotton, K. (2011). High-fidelity simulation debriefing in nursing education: A literature review. *Clinical Simulation in Nursing.* **7** (5), e161–e168. doi:10.1016/j.ecns.2011.02.001.

Raemer, D., Anderson, M., Cheng, A., Fanning, R., Nadkarni, V. & Savoldelli, G. (2011). Research regarding debriefing as part of the learning process. *Simulation in Healthcare.* **6**, S52–S57.

Rudolph, J.W., Simon, R., Rivard, P., Dufresne, R.L. & Raemer, D.B. (2007). Debriefing with good judgment: combining rigorous feedback with genuine inquiry. *Anesthesiology Clinics.* **25**, 361–376.

Rudolph, J.W., Simon, R., Dufresne, R.L. & Raemer, D.B. (2006). There's no such thing as 'nonjudgmental' debriefing: A theory and method for debriefing with good judgment. *Simulation in Healthcare.* **1**, 49–55.

Simon, R., Raemer, D.B. & Rudolph, J.W. (2009). *Debriefing Assessment for Simulation in Healthcare (DASH) – rater version.* Cambridge, MA: Centre for Medical Simulation.

Warrick, D., Hunsaken, P.L., Cook, C.W. & Altman, S. (1979). Debriefing experiential learning exercises. *Journal of Experiential Learning Simulation.* **1**, 91–100.

Wickers, M.P. (2010). Establishing the climate for a successful debriefing. *Clinical Simulation in Nursing.* **6**, e83–e86. doi: 10.1016/j.ecns.2009.06.003.

Chapter 6

Simulation for the inter-professional team

Key points

- Inter-professional education can improve team working, communication and patient safety
- Inter-professional simulation education also helps the development of human factor awareness
- There is often no inter-professional natural feedback or development of human factor and team working skills for healthcare teams

The importance of healthcare simulation in improving patient safety through the development of team skills in the multi-professional team is being increasingly recognised, and it therefore merits its own chapter in this book.

The growth of IPE and IPSE

There is still a fixation, both at undergraduate and postgraduate level, on training staff to work on their own, rather than as members of a multi-professional team. Professor Salas in the US eloquently described this as the 'training of a team of experts rather than an expert team' (Burke *et al.* 2004). Healthcare simulation allows us to work with these multi-professional teams, to develop an understanding of the limitations of human behaviour, how teams interact and the different professional roles. As individual roles in healthcare advance into more advanced roles, with further blurring of professional boundaries, this team training in the simulated learning environment becomes ever more important.

In healthcare, there has been growing interest in inter-professional education (IPE), where different professions learn together. Inter-professional education is defined as 'occasions when two or more professions learn from and about each other to improve collaboration and quality of care' (CAIPE 2002). This differentiates it from multi-professional learning, where different professional groups are present but do not learn from and about each other. When simulation is used in this process, it is referred to as inter-professional simulation based education (IPSE) (Gough 2012).

The interest in IPE was initially triggered by the publication of the Institute of Medicine's *To Err is Human* report (IOM 1999), which highlighted the need to improve patient safety through various mechanisms, including developing a 'culture of safety' in healthcare and team training. Within the UK, the Department of Health has supported 'common learning' and the need for more human factor training (Donaldson 2009).

Advantages and issues relating to IPE and IPSE

Undergraduate barriers to IPSE sessions include the physical size of the larger multi-professional group, difficulty in scheduling different student groups, associated cost of the sessions and the need to have a simulation competent multi-professional faculty (Gough *et al.* 2012). However, simulation in the hospital environment can overcome some of these issues, as all the learners are in practice placement together.

Although IPE is becoming more embedded in medical and nursing undergraduate curricula, it is still lacking within certain groups (*ibid.*). Often, the learners are only presented with a minimum number of sessions and there is a lack of scope to continue to develop team skills as an undergraduate or qualified individual. Within clinical practice, postgraduate IPE is not established and there are few, if any, team development opportunities. This often means that staff members do not develop an awareness of the roles of other professionals, which may also impede development of their own professional identity. In practice, the only feedback as to the effectiveness of the multi-professional team is often patient outcome, which may not be a reliable indicator of team working/team effectiveness, particularly with the acutely ill patient. The introduction of suitable team training can develop multi-professional team working and communication. Furthermore, it can identify situations where errors are more likely and offer strategies to avoid them. Repeated exposure to such learning opportunities allows such skills and behaviours to be identified, developed and learnt experientially (Donaldson 2009). There may also be an opportunity for some of the tools developed for use in debriefing the simulated scenarios to be used in actual clinical events to encourage debriefing and further team development.

Furthermore, it needs to be recognised that we do not currently train undergraduates or postgraduates to work together as a multi-professional team. Awareness of leadership, team working, communication and situational awareness is therefore developed on an inconsistent, ad hoc basis. Yet lack of these human factor (or non-technical) skills has been highlighted as the root cause in up to 70% of patient harm events. IPSE therefore has the potential to improve knowledge of other professional groups as well as inter-professional communication (*ibid.*) and ultimately patient safety.

Table 6.1: **Advantages and issues relating to IPSE**

Advantages	**Issues**
Learning together to work together	Groups are larger
Real team hierarchy	Difficult to release certain groups from practice
Allows natural escalation of care	Need a credible facilitator or several facilitators from different backgrounds
Develops human factor awareness	Learning outcomes need to be more generic and focused on patient safety

Running a dedicated simulation session in a learning environment will always be an approximation to the real clinical world. It will never be entirely real – the people participating often will not know each other, may work on different ward areas or specialties, and are often only from selected groups. Facilitating an event in practice is the opposite of this. The people present are part of the actual team and will encompass all the extended team members, including the lower grades and supporting specialties. Wherever training is located, there are certain difficulties that need to be anticipated when running IPSE events.

Learning outcomes in IPE and IPSE

Learning outcomes need to be very generic to allow a broad scope of practice for different professional groups. For example, with an asthma simulation, there is no point in saying 'assess the breathing and blood gas results' if the healthcare assistants and nurses present would not normally perform these tasks. However, if the first expected action is to 'effectively assess and respond to the deteriorating asthmatic patient', this allows all professional groups to respond appropriately within their scope of practice.

Barriers to wider use of IPE and IPSE

Specific treatments may also be initiated by different groups, depending on local policy. The facilitator/s therefore need to be aware of and conversant with the variable scope of practice relating to different grades and professional roles. Ideally, the faculty will be multi-professional and focused on inter-professional education.

Suzanne Gough and her colleagues demonstrated that undergraduate IPSE sessions were typically run for medical and nursing staff and it was less common to find other professions involved, or a larger number of professional groups represented (Gough *et al.* 2012). As the number of professionals increases, the total size of the cohort expands, requiring additional sessions. The faculty size also increases in line with the need to have faculty representing the different groups.

It is often not possible to get additional training made mandatory, at least in the initial development stages. This will make it harder to get certain staff released from practice. You may find one professional group is released but another is not, and this sometimes requires individual negotiation with ward/department managers. Here, the governance department can be a useful ally, especially if it becomes apparent that wards that actively engage in IPSE have a demonstrable reduction in patient safety incidents and litigation.

Issues that are unique to IPSE

Roles

As always, it is important to keep the roles of the learners in the simulation aligned to what they actually are in practice. The hierarchy within the group will dictate that more junior staff will naturally hand over, and expect more senior staff to run the situation. If the candidates are from multiple grades and professions, this may automatically limit the role of the junior staff. This can be addressed by phasing in the attendance of the team. Initially, two junior members arrive and assess the patient, calling for help when they naturally would. In this manner, the team can arrive in sequence, allowing individual staff to work to the limit of their practice before more senior staff take over. Conversely, running a session for a group of the same grade/profession can also present problems, as there will be no one to perform more junior tasks or more senior ones. Whilst it is possible for a facilitator to provide some senior direction, it can be challenging to keep the scenario realistic. We do not want to give the message that the learners can attempt activities that are outside their scope of practice. This is one element that needs to be considered in depth during the scenario development stage.

Learning outcomes

Again, learning outcomes should be generic where possible. For example, 'respond appropriately to the airway obstruction'. Team learning outcomes may be better suited to the inter-professional group (for example, 'communicate effectively as a team'). These could perhaps be supplemented by profession-specific learning outcomes. For example, the junior doctor would be expected to interpret the arterial blood gas result for the patient.

Faculty

As already mentioned, it will be necessary to increase the number of faculty to reflect the increased number of sessions and the diverse backgrounds of the learners. In addition, more novice faculty will need to develop skills in facilitating IPSE. They will also have to devote some time to collaborative working in order to identify common core elements and areas not shared by different professional groups (Baily *et al.* 2012). The scenarios may require adaptation and learning outcomes will have to be made more generic. Facilitating a hierarchical group, which contains varying cultural, social and clinical practices, will also require development of the faculty team. Baily and his colleagues pointed out that where such multi-professional training was suddenly established, it could highlight differences in simulation practices and create a need for a more standardised approach (*ibid.*).

Funding

Funding may also be an issue, as certain faculty may only be funded for education linked to specific staff groups. In addition, certain learners may have clear funding streams, while others will be less transparent. Where local facilities are not available, there may be the requirement to commission sessions for external providers or to establish a local facility, both of which will have cost implications. Often, some flexibility is required to resolve these issues and work collaboratively.

There is further discussion of using IPSE in Chapter 8 (on simulation in the clinical area) and Chapter 10 (on simulation and resuscitation training).

References

Baily, L., Bar-on, M., Yucha, C. & Snyder, S.J. (2012). Six challenges encountered in the opening of a multi-institutional, inter-professional simulation centre. *Clinical Simulation in Nursing.* In press. doi:10.1016/j.ecns.2011.12.002.

Burke, C., Salas, E., Wilson-Donnelly, K. & Priest, H. (2004). How to turn a team of experts into an expert medical team; guidance from the aviation and military communities. *Quality and Safety in Health Care.* **13** (Suppl 1), i96–i104.

Centre for the Advancement of Inter-Professional Education. (2002). *Inter-professional education – a definition.* London: CAIPE. Retrieved from http://www.caipe.org.uk/resources/

Donaldson, L. (2009). *Safer medical practice: machines, manikins and polo mints. 150 years of the annual report of the Chief Medical Officer: on the state of public health 2008.* London: Department of Health, HMSO.

Gough, S., Hellaby, M., Jones, N. & MacKinnon, R. (2012). A review of undergraduate inter-professional simulation-based education. *Collegian.* **19** (3), 153–70.

Institute of Medicine. (1999). *To Err is Human: Building a safer health system.* Institute of Medicine, National Academy of Sciences.

Chapter 7

Simulation in a dedicated simulation area

Key points

- A dedicated simulation area forms a controlled environment
- Such an area will have dedicated staff, supported by a wider faculty
- The cost of developing and running such an area should not be underestimated
- Such an area should mimic actual clinical areas
- Ex-clinical areas can be converted into simulation areas to reduce costs
- An organised group needs to run the area and engage with the organisation

Simulation in a dedicated teaching area can provide an ideal safe area for learning – away from the distractions of the clinical area (Gaba 2004), in what has been described as a 'controlled environment where learners can make, detect and correct patient care errors without negative consequences' (Issenberg 2005). The learners will often attend such a session without work colleagues or peers, and will thus feel more able to participate and ask questions (Møller *et al.* 2012).

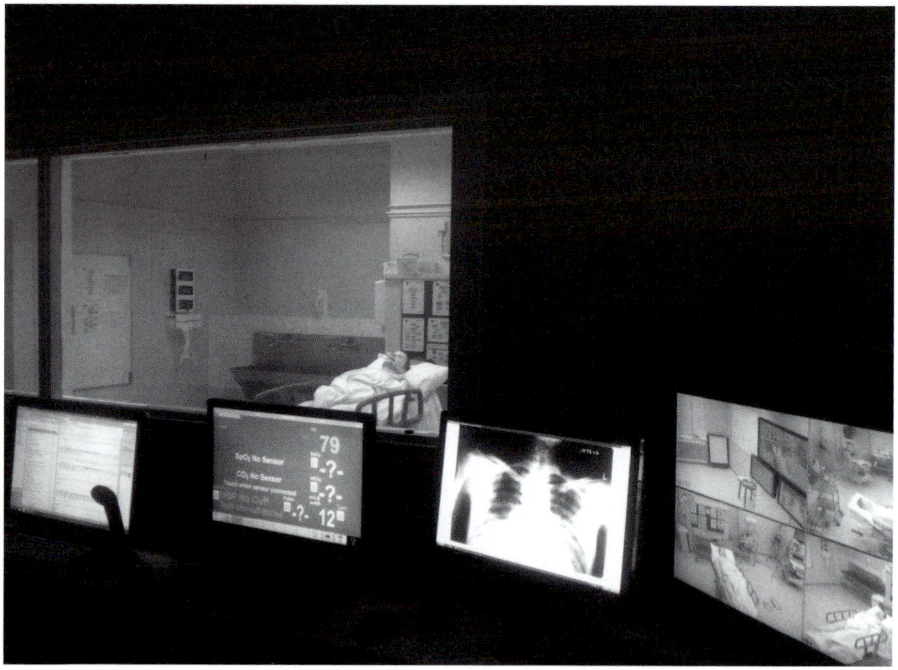

Figure 7.1

The simulation area viewed from the control room at North Manchester General Hospital

What faculty will work within the area?

Some staff will work in this area all the time, and others will come in to assist with specific sessions as required. These assisting faculty members will often be senior nursing, medical and other staff, who will bring their particular professional knowledge and be supported by the full-time staff. Some of these supporting staff will have teaching (and possibly simulation) roles written into their job descriptions, but some extra staff will not. If they are needed to make a regular commitment, it may be necessary to make some type of formal arrangement with the individual or their department in order to avoid simply relying on goodwill.

The physical area

A controlled simulation environment normally consists of at least one area for simulation and debriefing, often with additional simulation areas and space for lectures or practical skills sessions. There may also be a need for administrative and technical support staff, not only to assist with simulation technology but also to provide information technology (IT) and audio-visual (AV) support for presentations.

A technician can help to prevent damage to expensive AV and simulation equipment through inadvertent misuse by inexperienced faculty. It is often not recognised that time-consuming tasks such as setting up equipment and basic fault-finding would be better performed by a technician than by faculty members. Not all teaching staff will be confident in running the manikin and associated equipment. Having a trained technician to assist in this role will enable more staff, with different spheres of expertise, to facilitate simulation sessions. The presence of administrative and technical support staff will therefore aid coordination and allow for a larger throughput of users.

A dedicated teaching area, with a regular flow of learners and courses, also provides an ideal location in which to carry out further simulation research. There may be funding for local education fellows and learners on education courses to be based at the simulation centre, with suitable supervision from the senior faculty. This work can help to develop new areas of simulation activity, validate existing activity, and raise the profile of simulation within the organisation.

What kind of sessions can be run?

A wide variety of learning sessions can be run in such an area. For example, they may include undergraduate Objectively Structured Clinical Examination (OSCE) practice, resuscitation training, simulation sessions – indeed any sessions that you can think of, and possibly some that you can't! Imagine a mock ward area in which student radiographers can practise manoeuvring X-ray machines around typical ward obstacles, or an area to lay out 'risks', or practise evacuation training, or moving and handling training. The list goes on. Longer sessions can be facilitated when using a dedicated area (rather than running sessions in-situ). For example, planned sessions can be run for a whole day, incorporating a number of connected scenarios, that will continually develop staff.

Where should the area be located?

There are several options when deciding where to locate a dedicated simulation area. The final decision will depend on numerous factors, including availability of a location, funding, expected use and the time required to establish the facility. In some situations, the best solution will be to have a self-contained, bespoke area that has been built specifically for the purpose. This allows every aspect to be considered and planned in advance. It also means that learning in the area can be maximised, and will include consideration of the flow of learners and faculty through the area. Horley suggests that it is beneficial to keep a 'back of house area' in which faculty and technical staff can move around without disturbing or confusing the learners (Horley 2008). However, the cost of such a project should not be underestimated. Even with the use of an existing building, the budget may run into several hundred thousand pounds. The continuing maintenance and staffing costs also need to be considered.

What does such an area consist of?

The minimum requirements for a dedicated simulation area will include the simulation area itself, with an attached control room, debriefing area, toilets and storage areas. The storage requirements are often underestimated, as a considerable number of props, training aids and manikins may be needed.

The control room is often adjacent to the simulation area, and normally has a one-way mirror. The control room also houses all the computer equipment needed to control the manikin, as well as any AV equipment. In addition, there will often be a phone that connects the simulation area to the control room so the learners can phone for help and advice, and control room staff can simulate other hospital departments phoning with relevant information. There may be a dedicated computer and monitor in the room, where electronic resources such as ECGs, chest X-rays and blood results can be produced. It is useful if the control room can be entered externally from the simulation area, to allow faculty to come and go as required. There needs to be sufficient space for several people to work, and the room will require some soundproofing. The debriefing room is an informal area with AV equipment, where the learners are taken following the scenario. This room often has chairs set out in a circle or semicircle.

Equipping the simulation area

Rather than constructing a dedicated simulation area, a more achievable solution may be to utilise a redundant clinical area, and this will have the additional advantage of already looking like a realistic practice area! Many organisations invest in education areas and then retrofit the equipment to simulate a clinical area. Think of all the features you would need to simulate a realistic ward – beds, tables, chairs, commodes, patient lockers, a nurse call system, phones, medical gas supply, suction, and so on. Although these 'props' can often be left out, their presence will certainly increase the environmental fidelity and learner 'buy-in' during the session. Remember, our aim is to recreate the actual environment as accurately as possible, rather than creating a modified reality. If the natural first response on a ward, following a patient-based emergency, is to pull the nurse alarm, then this should be the same in our simulation area – or we risk drilling this response out of learners.

As well as reinforcing existing behaviours, a working clinical area may also identify gaps in knowledge. I remember once working with a group of medical students and discovering that, whilst they could describe a myriad of indications for oxygen therapy, none of the group could use an oxygen flowmeter. This would have remained undiscovered if working oxygen regulators and medical gases had not been available.

Sometimes older equipment, which is no longer serviceable for patient use, can be utilised in the simulation area. However, it is also important to include current equipment, both to maintain environmental fidelity and also as the use of current equipment may be included in the learning outcomes – for instance, using a syringe driver that is the same type as the one used on the ward.

Other issues affecting simulation area design and location

When designing the simulation area, remember that it needs to be in the context that the learner normally works in. For example, is it a good idea to set up an area as a critical care facility if the majority of the Trust staff work in a ward environment? It may be worth having an area with more than one bed – a ward bay, for example. Whilst the majority of scenarios will run with one manikin, there may be times when several could be utilised (or indeed the whole bay, to facilitate a ward scenario), remembering again that our simulated patients do not always have to be manikins. It's often advantageous to have a degree of flexibility so, with a quick change of equipment, the area could be a ward area, critical care or maternity area, for example.

There are some drawbacks to using an ex-clinical area for education. Firstly, circumstances may change and you could lose the area if it has to be used by real patients. There may then be issues around having equipment in the area that is out of date or not fully functional. However, with the necessary managerial support (and if you are able to prove that it is an effective, useful area), these risks can be mitigated. Often, the more you engage with the governance department, the greater the strategic support. Because of this, it is useful to make efforts to demonstrate how simulation sessions can address local issues, prevent incidents, and improve patient care and safety. All this should help to reduce the chances of suddenly losing your education area. There will also be some inevitable costs involved in converting the area into a suitable teaching area – for instance, providing IT infrastructure, computers and presentation equipment, as well as increased storage and office space.

In some ways, in-situ training in a real practice environment can be seen as the best option for team training because it uses the actual team, with all the distractions of the real clinical area (Bradley 2006). However, it would clearly be difficult to use a real setting for anything but very short sessions. Also, although learners are used to working in established teams, these teams often have new temporary members or have to work with other, unknown teams. This makes the inclusion of strangers contextually normal for sessions run in a simulation area.

A training area away from clinical pressures is an ideal environment in which to run programmes for new staff, clinical skills training and also inter-professional education (IPE), including sessions based on human factors and patient safety. Team sessions can focus on role development, rather than on how individuals work together. Without the pressures of interacting with 'real' patients, staff can reflect not only on their own professional roles but also on the roles of other professional groups, which can often help to contextualise and develop their perception of their own role.

Following one IPE session, a member of the nursing staff admitted that, despite having worked alongside one of the medical staff for a considerable period of time, she had learnt a great deal that day about the other person's role and now understood why doctors undertook certain actions. This is inter-professional education in practice! Imagine having groups of newly qualified doctors working in a simulated ward area as part of a multidisciplinary team induction, prior to being released onto the wards with real patients. Think of the advantages of including medicine management, communication, team work and developing professional identity in their training, and it seems clear that it would be quite easy to develop a course that would improve patient safety while also reducing stress for these relatively inexperienced doctors.

The use of video

Sessions run in a dedicated simulation area will often be more structured and planned, as you will have the advantage of knowing the professional groups of the candidates before they arrive, and in some instances may be able to prescribe the skill mix of the groups. It is more likely that video-assisted debriefing will be used, though this will again depend on the available funding and supporting faculty expertise.

Video will be overtly used and discussed, as part of the introduction to the area and session. It is important to clearly explain the reasons for the use of video – not only for the consent process but also to further engage the learners and create a safe environment where they feel they can express their feelings, concerns and questions without any repercussions. It is also important to state what will happen to the video recordings after the session. Most sessions will delete them and keep no permanent record.

Be aware, though, that the use of video will add another degree of complexity. Firstly, there is the need to learn how to operate and record the video, and secondly a decision has to be made about how to incorporate the video within the debriefing event. There are different ways of using video recordings. One very basic way is simply to show it live in a room nearby. This so-called 'streaming' allows the rest of the learners to view what is happening while it happens. This can become a more active task if the viewing learners are asked to monitor certain activities such as leadership or communication. The video clip may then not be used in any further debriefing.

Another option is to play the entire video recording at the beginning of the debriefing, or play a short section, stop and discuss, then play again. Obviously this is not a very effective use of time. A more advanced option is to use dedicated computer software to tag (mark) the required clips. Some software allows you to construct assessment frameworks and embed video collection automatically within the frameworks. The videos can now be selected at will, or edited into a stream of important, relevant events. This step may also assist in the gathering of data for research and faculty audits or development. However, it will require extra training for faculty members and is perhaps best suited to situations where there is a dedicated, full-time faculty. It is important that the debriefing session is not led by the video playback facility, but rather that the video facility is used to enhance the educational process of the debriefing.

Who runs the simulation area?

It is vital for a particular individual to have ownership or control of the simulation area. As the area will be used by many different people, there needs to be a designated person to oversee its use, and take responsibility for organising maintenance, arranging security and ordering equipment. The DH TEL framework (DH 2011) also identifies the need to have, not only this lead individual, but a group with clear aims, including a statement as to which learners the simulation resource is for. Such a group should ideally include medical, nursing and allied healthcare professional representatives, as well as leads from relevant departments. Some meetings may also be open to patient and learner representatives.

It is important for this group to coordinate simulation across the entire organisation. This will ensure that simulation is holistic and cohesive, with equity of access and reinforcement of key principles. It should also mean that the quality assurance process and faculty development can extend across the whole organisation. If the organisation does not understand the importance and potential benefits of the training, there may be some reluctance to release busy staff from ward areas and continue funding. The group running the simulation area will therefore have to engage with the organisation. For instance, discussions with the clinical governance department may yield opportunities for the simulated area to demonstrate best practice and equipment handling, following incidents that have occurred around the hospital. It could thus be part of a strategy to prevent similar occasions arising again.

These issues need not be overt, overly time-consuming or detract from session learning outcomes. An example would be an incident involving an item of equipment that was wrongly assembled – for instance, wall-mounted suction. If a scenario involved the use of suction, then the liner could be changed at the end of the scenario, thus demonstrating key points. This example shows how the faculty members need to be conversant with recent events in the organisation, as well as being aware of a wide range of local and national policies. As part of the group's evaluation of learning events, an audit of the area's utilisation should be included, to provide ongoing evidence of the usefulness of the area.

The ability to run formal, planned simulation sessions over a day or two is very important. In the next chapter, we will look at how running a simulation session in a clinical practice setting requires a very different approach.

References

Bradley, P. (2006). The history of simulation in medical education and possible future directions. *Medical Education*. **40**, 254–62.

Department of Health. (2011). *A framework for technology enhanced learning*. London: Crown Copyright.

Gaba, D. (2004). The future vision of simulation in health care. *Quality and Safety in Health Care*. **13**, i2–i10.

Horley, R. (2008). Simulation and skill centre design, in R.H. Riley (ed.) *Manual of Simulation in Healthcare*. Oxford: Oxford University Press.

Issenberg, S.B., McGaghie, W.C., Petrusa, E.R., Gordon, D.L., & Scalese, R.J. (2005). Features and uses of high-fidelity medical simulations that lead to effective learning: a BEME systematic review. *Medical Teacher*. **27** (1), 10–28.

Møller, T.P., Østergaard, D. & Lippert, A. (2012). Facts and fiction – Training centres or in situ. *Trends in Anaesthesia and Critical Care*. **2** (4), 74–9.

Chapter 8

Simulation in the clinical area

Key points

- In-situ simulation can reinforce and develop skills learned in more formal sessions
- It can be used for a number of purposes
- It has the utmost reality because it uses the actual environment and the actual team
- It can help to detect latent organisational system risks
- It can be used to develop human factor awareness in the actual clinical teams
- All simulation activity needs to be coordinated and quality-assured

Simulation in the actual clinical environment, or in-situ simulation, can present certain challenges and risks, which need to be mitigated. However, it can also be a very rewarding experience for all concerned. It has the potential to develop and stimulate cultural and organisational change (Hamman *et al.* 2007), developing team working, human factor awareness and improving patient safety (Riley *et al.* 2011). This type of simulation, probably more than any other, is likely to see expansion in the future. In my view, simulation in a dedicated simulation area will always remain the cornerstone of simulated learning but, in a large organisation, the capacity of such a resource is rapidly reached. In-situ simulation, in contrast, offers a real opportunity to reinforce and develop this type of formal training exponentially across a whole organisation, whilst simultaneously identifying latent embedded errors.

On the other hand, it is worth mentioning at the outset that there will be a high level of cancelled sessions. These sessions are also labour-intensive for faculty members, in terms of planning and facilitation. Equipment needs to be transferred, set up and prepared. Time also has to be spent on negotiating access with senior staff and identifying any local site-specific learning needs.

What can in-situ simulation be used for?

In-situ simulation can potentially be used to develop an inter-professional team with individuals but can also be employed to detect latent (organisational) errors. In addition, in-situ simulation may be used to test new procedures, changes in service, or policies to engage with staff. Scenarios can also involve different areas and departmental boundaries to look at difficulties in patient transfer arrangements, such as the transfer of a patient on a balloon pump from a catheter lab to a cardiac theatre.

Simulation in practice can be used to rehearse a planned event or difficult procedure, allowing staff to confirm their roles and actions and plan for emergency, unexpected events. There is also some evidence of the benefit of recreating actual incidents (either in practice or in a dedicated area) as part of the process of determining why a situation developed and how it could have been prevented. Personally, I think these sessions would need to be handled very sensitively and are more like a formal counselling session requiring specialist skills, and it would be easy for them to be seen as a punitive measure. But, with the correct support and faculty, it could be a useful exercise.

Different modalities of in-situ training

Simulation in the practice environment tends to fall into one of three categories: an established local faculty that runs regular sessions in a specific ward or department; an external (to the area) faculty that runs regular sessions in a specific ward or department; or a faculty that runs sessions across the entire institution. In-situ simulation can either be run as an announced planned event or, at the other end of the spectrum, as a planned but unannounced emergency drill (Walker *et al.* 2012). More information on facilitating emergency drills in practice is included in Chapter 10 (on simulation and resuscitation training).

Table 8.1: **Modalities of in-situ training and their common uses**

Modality	Faculty	Common uses
In-situ regular department/ ward-based	Local	• Induction of new staff • Introduction of new equipment • Human factor development • Skills training • Rehearsal of planned event • Prevention of skills fade • Response to incident • Identification of latent/organisational errors • Reinforcing of formal simulation sessions
In-situ department/ ward-based programme	Organisational simulation faculty	• Recreation of incident • Remedial simulation activity • Identification of latent/organisational errors • Reinforcing of formal simulation sessions
In-situ across whole organisation	Organisational simulation faculty	• Identification of latent/organisational errors • Prevention of skill degradation in the responding team • Reinforcing of formal simulation sessions • Human factor development for teams that respond across institution • Testing of new policies and procedures for usability

From the above table, it can be seen that there are some common themes and a degree of crossover, although certain modalities are better suited to some types of in-situ simulation than others and also represent the best use of the faculty's limited time. It is important that local simulation staff are supported and allowed to develop their competence in simulation and reinforce any wider training. All too often, these local champions work in isolation but they should be recognised, supported and developed as part of the organisation's cohesive approach to simulation. There are some possible drawbacks in using local faculty, including the question of whether and how often they can be released from other duties, their degree of competence in using simulation as a learning tool, and issues around debriefing peers and colleagues (Møller *et al.* 2012). However, as simulation expands, there is a need to engage and utilise these local experts and assist them, whilst always aligning their activity to local standards and those of the Department of Health TEL framework (DH 2011).

Advantages of in-situ simulation

Practice simulation is not designed to replace planned simulation sessions run in a dedicated simulation area but it can reinforce these sessions, prevent skills degradation, further develop certain skills, and be more inclusive than more formal sessions. Perhaps most importantly, in-situ simulation has far more benefit than dedicated simulation area sessions in identifying underlying, embedded latent system issues that can potentially lead to patient harm events, whether these are derived from policy/procedure, equipment or system processes (Riley 2011). It also has the potential to identify deliberate 'work arounds', where parts of standard practice or protocols are deliberately omitted, or active breaches (Riley 2011) that may have become embedded within the clinical area.

In-situ simulation offers the chance to teach learners in an environment with the highest possible environmental fidelity – their actual workplace, working in their normal teams and with their own equipment, and achieves technical, conceptual and emotional realism (Møller *et al.* 2012). Such training is always multidisciplinary and therefore aligned to instruction in human factor awareness and team working. It also highlights failures in situational awareness, shared mental model and communication (Riley 2011). William

Hamman and his colleagues suggest that the manikins used normally only present approximately 20% of the challenges faced by a team (Hamman 2007). In-situ training allows us to significantly increase this percentage. Furthermore, in-situ training has been described as particularly useful for simple skills training and training of short duration (Møller *et al.* 2012).

Characteristics of in-situ simulation

There are a variety of reasons why training in the clinical environment may be chosen. One of these is that it allows testing of systems and processes. It may also be run to provide team training in relatively short sessions, in order to minimise disruption caused by staff having to leave the clinical area. Finally, it may be run to address specific issues at a specific location, as the result of an incident or near miss – though, importantly, this will often be part of an overall strategy. However, simulation in practice should not routinely be used as a teaching tool, as it will require multiple visits and staff will not be focused on training.

Because of the brief duration of the sessions (due to releasability of staff), it is better to plan short visits to a particular area. With a focus on identifying latent errors, these sessions will not be expected to target every member of staff. It may also be advantageous to run some of the sessions during periods of the day other than just 9am–5pm, as this may identify specific issues relating to this time. It is also possible to incorporate an educational initiative to develop team working across an identified team. This may be particularly easy to facilitate if this team is mobile (for example, the adult cardiac arrest team), and sessions can be run in different areas to detect latent areas, while allowing the emergency team repeated exposure for team development. This will, however, involve a high degree of planning.

Because of the sometimes ad-hoc nature of in-situ training, learning outcomes need to be very generic. Generally, it is better to use team learning outcomes (as opposed to individual ones), as this will help to keep the outcomes broad enough to cover the different professional and non-professional groups who may be present. Local issues and clinical incidents or concerns should also be integrated into the sessions. For example, whilst doing an in-situ training session on an intensive therapy unit (ITU), it came to light that there had been issues with inotrope infusions not being checked by nursing staff following handover. A scenario was run in which a member of the faculty handed over the patient and the nor-adrenaline syringe driver was deliberately left nearly empty (whether this was detected or not was mentioned in the debriefing). This shows how patient safety issues can be embedded within the scenario almost in a covert manner. Over a period of time and after numerous revisits, the department could demonstrate that the majority of nursing staff had undergone the training and the risk of this error occurring again had thereby been reduced.

With in-situ simulation, the whole clinical team can participate in the training. It is rarely possible to release an entire clinical team for a simulation session in a dedicated learning area, and this means that the opportunity to reflect on specific issues with the in-situ team is lost. In addition, sessions run in a dedicated simulation area tend to be run primarily for qualified staff. Consequently, the team in practice is not the same size, consistency or skill mix as the team in training. In-situ training can be completely inclusive and utilise any person or profession who is in the area and willing to participate. For instance, we can include the healthcare assistants, porters, physiotherapists and other staff who are often not routinely involved in more formal sessions.

Ultimately it would be very labour-intensive to provide in-situ sessions for the whole workforce and it would also be very disruptive. Depending on the organisational logistics, it may only be possible to visit a particular practice area on one occasion during a programme lasting several years. Clearly, these sessions should not therefore be viewed as opportunities to teach staff about new equipment or procedures. Deficiencies in competence may be detected in certain individuals but how big an impact will that have on the running of a large ward or department? The real advantage of in-situ practice-based sessions is that they can reveal systemic problems. Explaining this clearly at the beginning of the session will remove some of the doubts of individuals who may still be viewing such a session as an assessment of their personal performance. For instance, let's say we identify a problem involving two similar-looking packaged emergency drugs that are stored next to each other, or difficulties in accessing a vital piece of equipment. If we resolve this type of issue, it could have a significant impact on patient care in the future. Indeed, it is very unusual to run an in-situ session and not discover one or more patient safety issues like this waiting to happen.

One way of highlighting the effectiveness and importance of in-situ simulation is to provide relevant groups in the organisation with documented evidence of the errors that have been detected, resolved and thus prevented from occurring again. This information is particularly powerful if it is placed in a common language of incidents. For instance, demonstrating that an in-situ simulation has prevented 20 level five events and 50 level four events will gain the attention of very senior staff. It is also important to give follow up feedback to the participants on identified and actioned issues to maintain and increase their engagement too.

Assessing the risks of in-situ simulation

Just as learning in practice can be an ad-hoc event, so can facilitating simulation in the practice environment. There are numerous practical issues to consider when using simulation in practice, the most important of which is the safety and welfare of patients on the ward area. One of the first priorities is therefore to carry out a robust risk assessment considering potential problems and ways to mitigate these risks.

Table 8.2: **Examples of risks and ways of mitigating them**

Potential risks	**Ways to mitigate risk**
There may be low staffing levels	Plan ahead, work with ward management
A clinical emergency may occur on the ward	Run the session during a high staff time, e.g. changeover or audit day
A clinical emergency may occur shortly before or during the session	If due to sickness or unplanned event, cancel session
Patients or relatives may get distressed	Cancel session
Use of actual clinical equipment, making it unavailable for real patients	Stop session immediately, and realise that a team is already assembled so they can respond instantly

The default position is to stop or cancel the session as soon as any issues arise. I cannot overstate the importance of ensuring that training is always run sensitively. The concerns of ward, medical and other staff must be listened to – and there should always be a low threshold for cancelling sessions. Some of the risks can be mitigated by working with senior staff to find the best time to facilitate the session. This may, for instance, be at a shift changeover, during an audit session or another quiet period.

Part of the risk assessment process should be to consider how to progress from identifying risks through simulations to implementing actual organisational change. Some of these actions may need to be immediate, and others will require careful consideration and the involvement of other groups and departments. Without this process, findings may end up getting lost in the system and never actioned. Realistically, this is something that will develop over a period of time. As the benefit of the simulations is revealed, interest in implementing their findings will increase.

Where to run in-situ simulation sessions

Some thought also needs to be given as to where to run in-situ simulations. This will partly depend on the learning outcomes and also on which areas are available for use. Ideally, these sessions will be held in a side room or an area that is away from the direct gaze of patients and visitors, and this is particularly important for the debriefing process. However, there may be times when contact with patients and visitors is unavoidable, because of available beds or the area layout. If training is undertaken in an area that is near actual patients, care should be taken to communicate to these individuals and their relatives what is happening.

Often, patients and visitors find such sessions very positive for patient care but there needs to be some sensitivity about choosing which scenarios to run. For example, introducing your manikin as Fred who has just had a hernia repair and collapsed, and seeing the patient in the next bed turning pale and looking down at his inguinal hernia scar, is probably best avoided!

When simulating patient emergencies, one of the advantages is that they can occur anywhere. A day room or even staff rest room can therefore be used – and having the flexibility to use different areas will reduce the chance of sessions being cancelled.

In-situ simulation assessment and debriefing

Assessment of candidates occurs continuously during the scenario, as already described in previous chapters. However, it is during the scenario that this data must be gathered. This should involve the use of frameworks developed as part of the scenario design process, and will need to incorporate an awareness of the different professional roles and grades in the scenario and their scope of practice.

As in simulation in the dedicated simulation area, video-assisted debriefing may be considered. However, there is a risk of accidentally videoing real patients, relatives or members of staff who have not consented to being filmed, and this may mean that it is easier to omit this step. If the session is videoed, this does make it possible to review the session and score individuals and the team more objectively. It may also provide useful information on areas of further work needed, and the effectiveness of the session. However, bear in mind that the restricted time candidates will have available often means a shorter scenario, with fewer learning outcomes. It may also lead to a condensed debriefing event, which is more a focused discussion on what went well and what didn't (Hamman *et al.* 2007).

References

Department of Health. (2011). *A Framework for Technology Enhanced Learning.* London: HMSO.

Hamman, W.R., Rutherford, W., Fuqua, W., Seiler, B., Beaubien, J.M., Rubinfeld, I., Lammers, R., Liang, B.A. & Riley, W. (2007). In-situ simulation®: Moving simulation to new levels of realism within healthcare organisations. *Proceedings of the 3rd Safety Across High Consequence Industries (SAHI) Conference, St. Louis University.*

Møller, T.P., Østergaard, D. & Lippert, A. (2012). Facts and fiction – Training centres or in situ. *Trends in Anaesthesia and Critical Care.* **2** (4), 174–9.

Riley, W., Lownik, E., Parrotta, C., Miller, K., & Davis, S. (2011). Creating high reliability teams in healthcare through in situ simulation training. *Administrative Sciences.* **1**, 14–31.

Walker, S.T., Sevdalis, N., McKay, A., Lambden, S., Gautama, S., Aggarwal, R. & Vincent, C. (2012). Unannounced in situ simulation: integrating training and clinical practice. *British Medical Journal Safety Quarterly.* 00, 1–5.

Chapter 9

Simulation in a virtual area

Key points

- Virtual simulation includes a range of activity and platforms
- Virtual worlds can be used for a variety of learning events
- Virtual simulation will often reinforce or introduce actual sessions
- The scenario process mirrors the actual one, except that the location can be fantastic
- IT infrastructure and networking problems can hamper the use of virtual worlds
- IT support should be provided for both learners and faculty members

Up to now, we have concentrated on simulation within a physical space. However, there is growing interest in extending simulations into virtual areas. Virtual simulation is not a new idea but it has increased in use and application recently. Virtual simulation can range from online sessions that simply present a photo with a brief explanation and several options to choose from, through to complex virtual worlds. Like actual simulation, virtual sessions can focus on knowledge, skills or behaviour.

How does virtual simulation work?

The most popular, open-source, three-dimensional virtual world program used for education is the Second Life platform (Warburton 2009), developed by Linden Lab. Second Life is an online virtual world and has no restrictions on access. Some people use it as a form of social interaction or leisure activity but this virtual community and infrastructure also has educational potential. Although loosely based on a multiplayer game, such a description is misleading, as there is no goal or game focus in Second Life (Aebersold *et al.* 2011). People can simply explore virtually, and use their virtual personalities (avatars) to interact with individuals who have similar interests, within communities. The Internet allows these worlds to be used as a common learning area. Avatars can meet, work and live, much as they do in the actual world. It is particularly useful at times when people are geographically remote from each other. Institutions, organisations and businesses can purchase virtual land and construct areas for staff, students and members of the public to use. Some areas in Second Life have been established purely for educational purposes, and the NHS uses some of these areas for learners and patients.

To access the virtual world, a program is installed on a computer. Once accessed, an avatar can be created and moved around the environment, controlled by the user's computer keyboard or drop-down menus. Avatars can walk, run or fly, and the teleport function can be used to travel between different islands or areas. Verbal communication is performed either by typing, with speech bubbles appearing, or by connecting a microphone to the computer and talking direct. It is interesting to note that, as in real life, non-verbal communication is automatically used – for instance, turning towards an individual you are talking to, even though this is not strictly necessary.

Some businesses use Second Life for meetings, as they find the interaction of the avatars is more natural than a telephone-based conference call.

What are the advantages of virtual simulation?

Simulation in a virtual area can offer many benefits. Firstly, it allows geographically disparate individuals to meet without physically travelling. For instance, a guest speaker can give a lecture for several different universities, or run education sessions on history-taking, communication, and other topics for several healthcare organisations.

Videos and presentations can be played within Second Life, and one of the benefits of the virtual environment is that we are not bound by health and safety, physical or economic restrictions. Having said that, it is important not just to use Second Life as a virtual classroom or to replicate actual areas (Molka-Danielsen & Linneman 2009). With a little imagination, it is possible, for example, to have a talk on the red blood cell whilst sitting in a red blood cell, or construct a team work scenario in which candidates go through a door and find themselves on a spaceship which the team has to resolve.

Learner and faculty avatars can interact with each other, and they can also interact with programmed mechatrons (computer-run avatars), as can other Second Life users or faculty acting as patients. In this way, Second Life simulation supports a broad approach to simulation in an immersive scenario (Aebersold *et al.* 2011).

How is a virtual simulation set up?

Planning, facilitating and evaluating a clinical scenario in Second Life requires exactly the same processes as running an actual scenario – establishing learning outcomes, designing a realistic and valid scenario, including measurement of actions and providing debriefing. Embedded quality assurance processes are important, and the session should conform to the TEL framework (DH 2011) as virtual simulation is a form of technology-enhanced learning. Just as in the real world ('First Life'), some of the group members may observe the session from a second virtual room.

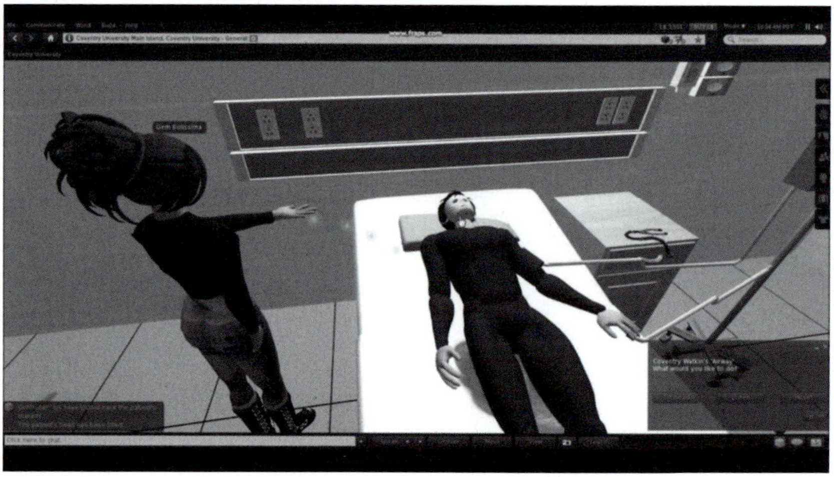

Figure 9.1
Deteriorating patient scenario run in Second Life on the North West Deanery Island

Figure 9.1 shows a demonstration that was put together for a conference where an OSCE could be run with a mechatron, to allow students to practise before an actual OSCE event.

Several emergency services have started using virtual reality programs for training, especially when developing command and control skills for larger emergencies that are difficult and costly to simulate in the real world. As with any type of education, the best strategy is to use a blended learning approach, rather than solely relying on one technique – so Second Life sessions can be used to augment and reinforce actual face-to-face sessions.

What are the obstacles to using virtual simulation?

There are some disadvantages to using virtual worlds for healthcare education and these include issues related to technology, time and culture (Warburton 2009).

Technical obstacles

The technical aspect of using the computer and program is often reported as being one of the main obstacles to using Second Life (Aebersold *et al.* 2011). The students will all require computers, of a relatively modern specification, with a broadband (high bandwidth) connection. The computers need to comply with a minimum specification, particularly in terms of processing power, video card performance, available RAM, firewall settings and Internet connectability (Molka-Danielsen & Linneman 2009).

There is another inherent issue with using Second Life within the NHS. Firstly, it is often generically classified as 'a game'. For this reason, it is often difficult to get IT departments to even discuss access. They may say that the site contravenes the organisation's IT policies, and many internal and external networks, including the NHS network, automatically block the use of Second Life. Secondly, even if access is allowed, the requirement for large bandwidth can hinder other patient applications and slow down Second Life. Therefore the best solution may be to encourage students to use it at home or in an education centre where they can access a dedicated external broadband connection. This may seem like circumventing the issue but does seem the easiest approach at the present time. Interestingly it has been reported that many learners also feel that Second Life is like a game, which can detract from their engagement with the session (Aebersold *et al.* 2011).

As with any new innovative learning tool, learners will need to familiarise themselves with the environment and how to use the program. Some type of induction into the environment will be required, and this will also require demonstrations on how to load and create an avatar as well as navigating, speaking and interacting with objects. This can be run as a face-to-face session or alternatively as an e-learning activity. Remember that the learners will have differing levels of familiarity with computers – thus a degree of technical support should be envisaged beyond that of just using the program.

In view of all this, Second Life is useful for learners who are involved in a programme of learning for a period of time, rather than as a one-off event. The learners need to be aware of the requirements for each session in advance. This is particularly important if they are expected to utilise their own computers from home, as they will need to be aware of minimum hardware and broadband specifications. Consideration will also have to be given to the possibility that some learners will not have access to this minimum. It is therefore suggested that, before the first meeting, learners access, install and create an avatar in Second Life (Molka-Danielsen & Linneman 2009) in order to save time in the session, allow problems to be resolved and concentrate on using the avatar.

In addition, Second Life resolution and rendering is not as high quality as a lot of modern video and computer-based games and is in fact slightly rudimentary, partly because of the way the environment is delivered on an as-needed basis. This is linked with the network signal delay (Aebersold *et al.* 2011), which often means that the environment is slow to change as the avatar moves from one area to another. These rendering issues may leave learners with a background in gaming feeling less engaged by Second Life than those without. The lack of resolution can affect the ability to perform certain tasks. For instance, cannulation would be difficult to perform, with the combination of reduced resolution and limited movements from the avatars. This is another reason why virtual simulation should not be used simply to recreate actual simulation. For example, there is no reason why certain tasks involved in cannulation cannot be tested – for instance, selection of appropriate equipment, patient consent, and so on. As mentioned earlier, the virtual simulation should be part of a blended approach to education, rather than the sole approach.

Time-related obstacles

The faculty will also need to become familiar with Second Life, and this raises the second barrier of time. Everything will take a long time to plan, validate and facilitate in Second Life (Warburton 2009). This is partly because it is often a new construct to the faculty, who have to spend time familiarising themselves with content and how to use the virtual world before contemplating using it as a teaching resource.

IT and computer issues will also affect the faculty. For example, there is often a requirement to source people who can build virtual environments. Because of this, Second Life use in the UK is often restricted to higher education institutions where there is a recognised group of individuals dedicated to Second Life learning as part of their role. It is unlikely that individuals within the NHS will have the time or expertise to set up a new, dedicated Second Life area themselves. However, learners may be able to gain access to established healthcare and university Second Life areas to augment their learning.

There are also some factors that need to be incorporated into the session. The faculty will often be at remote sites and will thus require some method of communicating with each other. In a real simulation, a faculty member would be able to talk quietly to a fellow facilitator or even use facial expressions to communicate. In a virtual simulation, this ability may need to be replaced by simultaneously running a chat room for faculty to communicate, off Second Life, about learner issues or problems. The learners will not, of course, be aware of this other communication channel.

Culture-related obstacles

The third barrier relates to culture. Second Life represents a new environment that can feel as if it is outside the 'safety zone', with a different etiquette and set of accepted behaviours (Warburton 2009). Some of these cultural concerns manifest themselves as security issues. For example, you cannot guarantee who is controlling the avatar. Thus you could potentially have someone else controlling one of the student avatars. This would be an especially worrying issue for any assessment process. Potential solutions may include asking candidates to attend a local area (still avoiding travel to a distant exam) or possibly using a webcam to confirm identity. Certain areas can be made secure, to stop non-invited people from attending. There is also some concern about some areas of these worlds being adult themed. However, as with all modes of communication and technology, there is always some potential for misuse and some degree of responsibility needs to be left with the learners. As part of the induction process, a documented Second Life code of conduct or expected behaviour should be discussed, which will often mirror actual world expectations.

References

Aebersold, M., Tschannen, D., Stephens, M., Anderson, P. & Lei, X. (2011). Second Life ®: A new strategy in educating nursing students. *Clinical Simulation in Nursing*. e1–e7.

Department of Health (2011). *A Framework for Technology Enhanced Learning*. London: HMSO.

Molka-Danielsen, J. & Linneman, L-C. (2009). Chapter 4: Sim creation and management for learning environments. In Molka-Danielson, J. & Deutschmann, M. (eds) *Learning and Teaching in the Virtual World of Second Life*. Trondheim, Norway: Tapir Academic Press.

Warburton, S. (2009). Second Life in higher education: Assessing the potential for and the barriers to deploying virtual worlds in learning and teaching. *British Journal of Educational Technology*. **40** (9), 414–26.

Chapter 10

Simulation and resuscitation training

Key points

- Simulation helps prevent degradation of resuscitation skills
- Simulation can identify latent and active errors
- A regular simulation programme will allow staff to develop human factor awareness
- Simulation should not be used as a resuscitation test
- A different skill set is required to plan, develop and run a simulated scenario
- Resuscitation officers should be encouraged to run simulation sessions effectively

Simulation can be used to help ensure that patients in cardiac arrest in hospital have appropriate high-quality resuscitation. It can also increase staff confidence and preparedness for emergencies (Banks 2012). In addition, regular training in recognising and managing the deteriorating patient may help prevent cardiac arrests. Simulation can be used in a number of ways, including increasing the effectiveness and realism of the simulation training process (including quality of debriefing) in existing courses, and establishing regular planned sessions within a dedicated simulation or practice environment (Andreatta *et al.* 2011, Banks 2012). Furthermore, it can be used in ad-hoc sessions throughout an organisation, with or without the activation of the relevant emergency team (adult or paediatric cardiac arrest, medical emergency, trauma, obstetric, etc.).

In addition, specific sessions may be planned following the expansion of services or physical layout to orientate staff (Sahu & Lata 2010), or test new systems and equipment (Walker *et al.* 2012). Such high-quality resuscitation education requires a multifaceted approach, integrating existing skill teaching, real-time feedback on performance, and briefing and debriefing education in non-technical (human factor) skills (Soar *et al.* 2010). Andersen and his colleagues found that various non-technical skills were required in resuscitation and these were: team leader experience, structured communication, mandatory use of cognitive aids, mutual performance monitoring and avoidance of task overload (Andersen *et al.* 2010).

Traditional resuscitation training and resuscitation simulation

Simulation is well established as a method of carrying out resuscitation training. However, it is often used within the rigid parameters and time constraints of external national courses. In these sessions, there tends to be a particular focus on the teaching of skills (Andersen *et al.* 2010) and subsequent testing of the candidate's knowledge. It has been suggested that resuscitation skills start to degrade rapidly following training. They usually require re-instruction within three to six months in order to maintain competence (Berden *et al.* 1993), as skills tend to degrade more quickly than knowledge (Yang *et al.* 2012). It is recognised that there is a lack of human factor and team development in such courses, and the lack of leadership development for medical staff (Hunziker *et al.* 2011) has been repeatedly raised.

This is not to imply that the current resuscitation training process is not fit for purpose. But there is certainly the potential for simulation to reinforce these sessions, prevent skill degradation, detect latent and active system errors, and develop team working. One large US study estimated (based on retrospective analysis) that resuscitation system errors occur in 40.4% of VF/ pulseless VT cardiac arrests and 26.8% of non-shockable arrests. This leads to decreased rates of return of spontaneous output, decreased survival to 24 hours and decreased survival to hospital discharge (Ornato *et al.* 2012). Simulation can work hand in hand with traditional resuscitation training but it does need to be appreciated that the simulation process is different from facilitating a resuscitation skills assessment. Skills such as debriefing and error detection can be developed and supported through suitable training, tools and mentoring from organisational staff running simulation sessions.

Table 10.1 (below) shows the main differences between a short traditional resuscitation course and a resuscitation simulation scenario.

Table 10.1: **Traditional resuscitation training versus simulation**

Item	Short resuscitation course	Simulation (formative)
Overall realism	Tends to be lower realism	Tends to be higher realism
Length of scenario	Relatively short	Can be longer
Length of debriefing	Short, concise feedback (to fit time constraints)	Longer debriefing sessions
Aim of scenario	To test/develop knowledge	To develop knowledge, skills or behaviours
Team provided	Standardised for test, random for others	As expected if using real team
Role of person running scenario	Instructor	Facilitator
Course design	Often external	Often internal

Running cardiac arrest drills

Cardiac arrest drills are staged cardiac arrest scenarios that are run for a number of reasons. They will typically activate the attendance of the relevant cardiac arrest team, often without them being aware that it is a drill. Such a drill can also be used as an opportunity for the ward staff to respond to a deteriorating patient scenario and may initially involve other organisational teaching staff such as members of the outreach team. One study reported that weekly in-situ simulations for a paediatric medical emergency team improved ward staff recognition and management of the deteriorating patient (Theilen *et al.* 2013). Another advantage is that the various teaching staff members are able to work together and reinforce each other's activity.

Clearly, there are pros and cons to running a cardiac arrest drill within a hospital. Although organising such a drill requires a lot of work, simulated practice has been shown to improve simulated outcomes. There is less evidence on the transferability of this effect to actual clinical practice (Sahu *et al.* 2010). However, in a widely reported study, Andreatta and her colleagues described a dose-related improvement in cardiac arrest outcome and staff confidence following a programme of cardiac arrest paediatric drills (Andreatta *et al.* 2011).

Table 10.2: **Advantages and disadvantages of running cardiac arrest drills**

	Positive issues	**Negative issues**
Activation of the hospital team	The attending team is the actual in-situ team and therefore a realistic size	Patient safety must be guaranteed; staff may be busy elsewhere
Ability to test adherence to standards	Compliance with relevant resuscitation standards can be assessed	There is sometimes an over-reliance on adherence to standards as the only key indicator
Ability to test systems	The organisation can now test scenarios in areas of concern proactively, to identify system issues	Needs to be an awareness that one particular result is not necessarily going to occur every time, in every place

Ability to access, reflect and develop team skills	Potential to develop team skills and encourage, promote reflective practice	These skills need to be facilitated by an individual with some knowledge of human factors and non-technical skills, guided by relevant tools and able to facilitate an objective debrief
Providing feedback to the whole resuscitation team	Debriefing allows reflection on the team's action and developing plans to develop this further in the future	May not be facilitated as a learning opportunity, in which case it will remain as an assessment event
Environmental fidelity	Ultimate in terms of reality, as equipment and layout are all real	Essential emergency equipment should not be depleted or made unavailable for actual patients' immediate need

During the planning stage of the drill, two tasks need to be undertaken. Firstly there must be a thorough and robust risk assessment, and secondly the sessions need to be widely advertised to staff to allow concerns to be addressed and initiate engagement at all levels.

The risk assessment process needs to be undertaken in order to mitigate risk, and it will need to look at the following questions:

1. Are the relevant staff available? Or are they dealing with an emergency?
2. What will happen if there is an emergency during the session?
3. What equipment can be used?
4. What issues will affect moving staff to a staged emergency?
5. When are the sessions going to be run? Will running them at different times (i.e. out of hours) change the risk levels?

Planning resuscitation simulations

One of the first considerations should be what we are going to assess and what our learning outcomes will be. To gain engagement from the staff, it is useful to shift the focus away from summative assessment of the technical process. Although positive feedback can be provided, it is important to remember that this is not a test. It is unrealistic to expect individuals who undertook a course several years before to perform as they did during the course. All the evidence and research shows that resuscitation skills degrade rapidly so testing an individual, in order to retest their skills, serves no purpose and only demotivates and disengages them from future training.

If we are going to assess technical compliance with current resuscitation practice, we will also need to define a safe standard. Clearly, not all providers will have the same level of resuscitation training, and it is not always clear what level of decay will translate to actual sub-optimal clinical performance that will affect patient outcomes (Yang *et al.* 2012), or even *if* a decay in simulated practice will necessarily correlate with a decay in clinical practice (Mosley *et al.* 2012).

When running these drills, the priority should be to identify latent and active errors, and further develop human factor awareness across the emergency response team. Regular drills will not typically be run in the same area; rather, they will target different locations. Again, the focus should therefore not be on testing and teaching, as we will only have access to a small percentage of staff in a particular area. In contrast, looking for system errors, and fixing them, can have an effect across the whole area and even institution.

Often the only feedback that the team has, following a cardiac arrest, is the patient outcome. However, this is a poor indicator of team performance, as it is recognised that prognosis is generally poor with cardiac arrests. With simulated cardiac arrests facilitator led debriefing can encourage reflective practice and team development.

Ultimately, this should occur even at a basic level, following actual clinical events as well. Performing drills in-situ allows us to use a real practice team, incorporating the local area staff as first responders. Compare this to the slightly sterile and forced team skill mix of formal resuscitation courses. In-situ sessions have great potential to assess, debrief and evolve the team skills of the team but they need to be carried out with considerable thought and care.

Frequency of sessions

The frequency of the event will be determined by the main reason for performing it. If it is being used to test systems and processes, it may not need to be performed with the same frequency as if it is being used to prevent skill degradation. Mosley and her colleagues point out that the exact frequency of such training is under-researched (Mosley *et al.* 2012). In addition, the frequency may partly depend on the pre- and post-course clinical experience of the learners (Yang *et al.* 2012). If a more formal training programme is being planned, the number of staff involved and the logistics of staffing will also affect the frequency. There will need to be a degree of redundancy built into the planning to allow for cancelled sessions.

Developing scenarios

Scenarios for use in practice or within a dedicated training area need to be worked out with thought and due process. A bad scenario will alienate candidates and will not promote simulation as a learning tool. Simply transferring an existing course testing scenario into a ward learning session is not advisable – it is not what it was designed or validated for. Chapters 1 to 4 (on planning, running and debriefing a scenario) will provide useful guidance on how to develop sessions that reflect local learning needs. It is also worth spending some time considering the cardiac arrest drill/mock code. As staff members are developing their skills experientially, each scenario does not have to be different. Indeed, allowing the learners to practise the same scenario again, at a later stage, enables them to implement some of the points discussed.

Do not be tempted to run an overly complicated scenario. Remember that these staff members are not on a course. They have not benefited from a day of teaching or had numerous previous sessions. We should therefore be careful not to set the level too high, with a scenario that is too complicated or too frightening. A simple scenario may just involve delivering the first shock. This will still provide plenty of debriefing information and will also allow more time for the debriefing.

Introducing sessions

With more formal simulation, we begin by reassuring the learners that this is a safe session, where they can speak freely of their concerns without repercussions. However, when the team arrives at a resuscitation scenario, there is no time for lengthy briefing and the introduction may simply be 'treat this manikin/person as if they were a real patient'. We will therefore need to spend time beforehand, in the run-up to the session, explaining its purpose and benefits. This is the time to gain staff engagement and explain that the role of the session is to develop the team and identify system issues. It is often reported that there is a degree of disengagement during the initial sessions, but (as word spreads about the benefits), faculty staff engagement will increase – to the point where departmental heads will be requesting their drill.

Assessment

As with any simulation session, time must be made available for the debriefing, and feedback from staff attending may be useful when planning future sessions. Once a training programme has been established, some of the assessment metrics can be included within debriefing following actual cardiac arrests, and the reflective process and staff development can thus be continued.

When assessing cardiac arrest technical management, we can perform an objective assessment by using our knowledge of the resuscitation algorithm as an assessment tool. We may even have this as a tick list. This objective assessment is also required for our non-technical or human factor assessment and some type of framework needs to be used, preferably with a previously validated metric or tool. This is particularly important for faculty members who are less experienced with assessing human factor (non-technical skills). Such tools as Objective Skill-based Clinical Assessment tool for Resuscitation (OSCAR) (Walker 2011) give exemplars of activity to guide assessment. This will enable the trained observer to rate the team. I say 'trained', as there needs to be a learning process with using these tools so that we develop rater-rater independence – that is to say, if one person assesses a team they should get the same results as another. Again, the focus in this assessment is on gathering data to support the debriefing. There may be a temptation to score individuals, but with little research available on the validation of such scoring, it is best avoided at this stage.

Engaging the wider organisation

It is, of course, vital to involve and engage other groups within the organisation, such as the resuscitation committee, resuscitation leads, clinical governance, medical director, medical education team, practice educators and outreach team. A clear documented list of the aims, benefits and risks of the simulation will be needed, as well as steps taken to mitigate the risks. The benefits will potentially include:

- Increased patient safety
- Decreased complaints and incidents
- Staff learning
- Better evaluation of resuscitation training
- Testing of new systems (e.g. new ward/building/shifts)
- Embedding/testing of new policies
- Benchmarking of internal standards (e.g. time of attendance of team).

Once permission and acknowledgement have been obtained, senior staff need to be informed about the sessions that are going to be held, and any concerns they may have should be addressed. A lot of potential issues will be resolved if senior medical staff buy into the rationale and reasons for running the sessions at the outset. When any identified issues have been resolved, a date and target area can be identified and the session run.

However, before the session is initiated and an actual emergency call is placed, it is vital to check whether there are any other acute events occurring in the area and/or involving the key players. It may be necessary to contact consultants and leads in acute areas to confirm that it is safe to proceed. Remember that some teams (such as trauma) may need to activate off-site individuals who may or may not be relevant to the scenario. Word-of-mouth rapidly spreads through an organisation about emergency calls so it may be necessary to warn certain areas (such as operating theatres) that there will be a planned drill in five minutes and they should not halt sending for patients, etc.

References

Andersen, P.O., Jensen, M.K., Lippert, A. & Østergaard, D. (2010). Identifying non-technical skills and barriers for improvement of teamwork in cardiac arrest teams. *Resuscitation*. **81**, 695–702.

Andreatta, P., Saxton, E., Thompson, M. & Annich, G. (2011). Simulation-based mock codes significantly correlate with improved patient cardiopulmonary arrest survival rates. *Pediatric Critical Care Medicine*. **12** (1), 22–38.

Banks, D. (2012). Optimizing patient resuscitation outcomes with simulation. *Nursing* **42** (3), 60–61.

Berden, H.J.J.M., Willems, F.F., Hendrick, J.M.A, Pijls, N.H.J. & Knape, J.T.A. (1993). How frequently should basic cardiopulmonary resuscitation training be repeated to maintain adequate skills? *British Medical Journal*. **306**, 1576–7.

Hunziker, S., Johansson, A.C., Tschan, F., Semmer, N., Rock, L., Howell, M.D. & Marsch, S. (2011). Teamwork and leadership in cardiopulmonary resuscitation. *Journal of American College of Cardiology*. **57**, 2381–8.

Mosley, C., Dewhurst, C., Molloy, S. & Shaw, B.N. (2012). What is the impact of structured resuscitation training on healthcare practitioners, their clients and the wider service? A BEME systematic review: BEME Guide No. 20. *Medical Teacher*. **34**, e349–85.

Ornato, J.P., Peberdy, M.A., Reid, R.D., Feeser, V.R. & Dhindsa, H.S. (2012). Impact of resuscitation system errors on survival from in-hospital cardiac arrest. *Resuscitation*. **83**, 63–9.

Sahu, S. & Lata, I. (2010). Simulation in resuscitation teaching and training, an evidence based practice review. *Journal of Emergency Trauma Shock*. **3** (4), 378–84.

Soar, J., Edelson, D.P., Perkins & G.D. (2010). Delivering high-quality cardiopulmonary resuscitation in-hospital. *Current Opinion in Critical Care*. **17**, 225–30.

Theilen, U., Leonard, P., Jones, P., Ardill, R., Weitz, J., Agrawal, D. & Simpson, D. (2013). Regular in situ simulation training of paediatric medical emergency team improves hospital response to deteriorating patients. *Resuscitation*. **84** (2), 218–22

Walker, S., Brett, S., McKay, A., Lambden, S., Vincent, C. & Sevdalis, N. (2011). Observational Skill-based Clinical Assessment Tool for Resuscitation (OSCAR): Development and validation. *Resuscitation*. **82** (7), 835–44.

Walker S.T., Brett S.J., McKay A., Aggarwal, R. & Vincent, C. (2012). The 'Resus:Station': the use of clinical simulations in a randomised crossover study to evaluate a novel resuscitation trolley. *Resuscitation*. **83**, 1374–80.

Yang, C-W., Yen, Z-S., McGowan, J.E., Chen, H.C., Chiang, W-C., Mancini, M.E., Soar, J., Lai, Mei-S. & Ma, M.H-M. (2012). A systematic review of the retention of adult advanced life support knowledge and skills in healthcare providers. *Resuscitation*. **83**, 1055–60.

Chapter 11

Simulation for assessment

Key points

- Simulation is most commonly used for formative assessment
- Exceptional rigour needs to be employed when using simulation for summative purposes
- It is essential to be able to demonstrate validity and reliability of assessment
- Competence in simulation does not equate to performance in practice
- Summative simulation assessment is best used as one of several different methods to make decisions
- There is limited evidence of the effectiveness of simulation as a summative tool but the evidence is expanding

Most simulations that occur within the hospital environment, perhaps with the exception of resuscitation training, are run as formative sessions and they are often enjoyable events for facilitator and learner alike. There will always be an element of assessment within each learning event but this is primarily to provide information for the debriefing, as opposed to deciding if the learner has passed or failed. When formal summative assessment *does* occur, simulation allows it to be performed in a standardised, planned and repeatable way, and to be recorded on video for later review (Weller *et al.* 2003). It is essential that assessment, even in formative sessions, is both valid and reliable. This is even more important for a summative assessment, where the stakes are higher and a decision one way or the other could result in a learner failing a course, module or year.

Although concerns have been expressed about using simulation for high-stakes summative assessment, there is some evidence of moderate levels of reliability and validity in optimal test conditions (Watterson 2008). Indeed, Holmboe and his colleagues suggest that there is now sufficient evidence and they recommend the wider piloting of simulation as part of the regulation of healthcare professionals (Holmboe *et al.* 2011).

Nevertheless, formal summative assessment is still a rarity, and needs to be planned and run even more robustly than formative assessment, as the facilitator could potentially be called to account if there are any doubts about the validity and reliability of the testing method. I have always been wary of questions such as, 'Do you mind just doing some scenarios with Doctor X? We have had some concerns and would like to know what you think.' This brings up a whole raft of issues: Who am I to assess this person? Do I understand what he should be able to do? Is this a knowledge, skills or behaviour issue? Am I happy to make high-stakes comments, or comments that could be used by others when making high-stakes decisions? Ultimately, how do we ensure that any assessment is always an objective, fair assessment?

Scenarios and assessment

The other question we need to examine is whether the specific scenario we generate is a valid and reliable test for this situation. Any scenarios for testing will be best developed on a national basis, in conjunction with the professional bodies of the individuals being tested. They will include clinical and educational experts and be validated by piloting with an appropriate number of people.

The scenarios have to be relevant to the particular individual at the time of training. This is particularly important when considering students and trainees – there is no point if we decide that the doctor concerned is not competent at a particular role and then discover that they are not supposed to be! The scenario will also have to be tested with a group not in difficulty (a control group) to demonstrate construct validity and to show that the metric can differentiate between the two groups.

The challenges of using simulation for assessment

There are several situations where simulation could be considered for use as a summative assessment tool, whether as part of an interview process, or to assess a struggling or failing learner, or to check that staff have certain competencies required for a particular stage or role. However, there are concerns around this process and the validity of using a simulated scenario. We need to ask, does what we see match what we would see in actual practice?

Unlike aircraft flight simulators, healthcare simulations lack a very high degree of realism. Whilst they have improved over recent years, they never appear entirely real. This is partly because the complexity of healthcare itself is difficult to recreate. For example, is it realistic to assess an individual on their own? Do we give the individual a team of obliging but mute helpers? Or do we have a realistic random team, with members floating in and out? If so, what size should the team be? Whilst there is almost certainly some degree of correlation between the scenario performance and practice performance, the precise degree of this correlation is less well understood. With all this in mind, we also need to be aware that if we use the scenario to assess competence, simulation competence will not equate to actual clinical performance competence. Whilst competence may predict performance, a competent practitioner may not be an effective one (Kak *et al.* 2001).

Personally, with all these questions and the need for a robust, fair process that can stand up to scrutiny, I would suggest this is not something that should be organised as a local activity. The assessment needs to be objective and standardised so that if a person passes at one site we would expect an identical result at another. This will also standardise the assessment process across the country, which will require some training for the facilitation faculty in the assessment process and metrics used (whether this training be online or face-to-face) and ongoing re-assessment to confirm that standards are being maintained.

Simulated high-stakes assessments have been described and used in medical education, especially for anaesthetists (Weller *et al.* 2003), though their use in other professional groups is less reported (Bensfield *et al.* 2012). As we move away from the 'see one, do one, teach one' model to that of learning on manikins rather than on patients, we are moving towards a more outcomes-based model, which will typically include some form of competency assessment. Despite criticisms of competency-based education as 'reductionist, narrow and simplistic', a competency framework that has been developed by relevant stakeholders can help transparently demonstrate consistent practice standards (Brownie *et al.* 2011). In addition, the accuracy of multiple simulated assessments will further increase their reliability (Murray 2004). With the dawn of medical revalidation, we will all probably become more involved with summative simulation assessments.

Though clinical skills and procedures can be assessed as part of a formative procedure – for instance, during an Objective Structured Clinical Examination (OSCE) – this will always be within a framework of current/best practice that is relevant to the individual. Often these tasks are assessed using a checklist. McKinley and colleagues reviewed 88 unique checklists and identified seven key themes. They found two of these key themes were only found in 32% and 51% of the checklists, respectively, and suggested that this might lead to inconsistency in the assessment of key competencies (McKinley *et al.* 2008). The very concept of competency raises concerns, as it is recognised that competency is multifaceted and includes knowledge, skills, abilities and traits (Kak *et al.* 2001), which makes it very complex to assess. Even with a relatively simple clinical skill, there can be controversy when a task is performed in a different order from the one expected, or if it is still safe but results in a fail, or such an unexpected event occurs that it is difficult to find an appropriate area in which to fail the candidate. Faculty members are often reluctant to fail students, especially when the evaluation reveals an area of ambiguity or imprecision (Wolf *et al.* 2011). Gaba and his colleagues also discuss the difficulty of assessing criteria that fluctuate over time (Gaba *et al.* 1998).

Validity and reliability

Validity and reliability in simulation can be further divided into various component parts, as shown in Table 11.1 (below).

Table 11.1: **Achieving validity and reliability in simulation**

Element	**Description**	**Example of how to achieve in simulation**
Content validity	Are the learning outcomes relevant and achievable by the learners?	Mapping content to curriculum or scope of practice. Awareness of knowledge, skills, framework requirements for specific roles
Construct validity	Does the assessment test what you want to? For example, assessing a candidate's ability to bake a cake may not prove they are good at assessing a patient	Linking the assessment to the learning outcomes, using validated assessment tools, or constructing one from national standards/guidelines
Predictive validity	Does the assessment reflect similar assessments or levels? For example, if the learner fails an assessment in resuscitation, do we find they have failed/struggled at a resuscitation in practice?	Comparing pass and fail rates of similar courses or assessments and concerns from practice
Rater-rater reliability	Do different faculty members achieve the same results for the same candidate?	Guidance on how to assess learners, guidance embedded on assessment form monitoring examiner results
Test/Retest reliability	If we tested the same individual twice, would we get the same result?	Programmed scenario with manikin that behaves in predicted way; use of validated assessments, piloting and trialing tests
Parallel forms reliability	Does the assessment reliably give similar results to another test with similar subject matter?	Comparing the simulation results to that of an OSCE or written exam; piloting with groups with known results to other test
Internal consistency	Does a learner of a particular grade show similar results across the whole scenario?	Piloting of scenario with suitable group and comparing results

Rater–rater reliability requires training and confirmation that it remains acceptable. Video-recorded scenarios can be retrospectively reviewed by expert raters and can then be used to standardise novice raters and verify a proportion of decisions, as part of a quality assurance programme. Studies have recommended a minimum of two trained raters to provide a reliable assessment (Weller *et al.* 2003) but there needs to be a policy in place for a situation in which the raters give differing scores.

Other variables that may affect assessment

Much more thought needs to be put into the choice of assessment tool used to assess the person, and the way in which the scenario is introduced. For instance, it would be unfair for a candidate to fail due to their unfamiliarity with the equipment provided or the manikin not working as expected. Indeed, I have seen medical students reacting poorly when the manikin they were used to was changed to a different make. This demonstrates the potential for contamination of the assessment results.

The scenario process should also be adequately explained, as should the roles of other people and faculty members. Remember, the learners may be more used to participating in formative scenarios, with instant feedback and debriefing, and may be thrown by a silent faculty. The addition of other team members introduces another variable, which is why these team roles are often played by faculty members. Ideally, the assessment tool should be a validated one – and validated for the specific group and situation. However, in practice, with certain groups, the validation of technical skills may arise from using agreed national standards, which are in effect validated standards. Also, remember that, whilst we may be able to suggest a causal relationship with competence in practice, we are still testing the candidate on a simulation and not a real situation. Simulations may be used to gather evidence about individuals who have difficulties or are struggling – but the simulation will only be one part of the information-gathering process, supplemented, for instance, by discussions and interviews. It is therefore more useful to see simulation as one of several methods to gather information on the candidate, rather than being used in isolation (Watterson 2008).

Simulation assessment debriefing

Debriefing of the testing scenario will often be brief, with maybe only a short time to ask any questions, partly for the faculty to gather further evidence. Often, there will be little need for a long debrief, and in some cases the use of weighted scoring sheets or retrospective scoring of videoed sessions may even mean that the faculty do not know the ultimate outcome of the assessment.

The simulation will often play a part in managing staff who are having difficulties. Unfortunately and realistically, the resolution may sometime include termination of employment or training. Objective, validated documentation of an individual's actions and abilities is therefore vital. In this situation, video feedback is particularly useful, as it provides incontrovertible physical evidence. Although termination is not a good outcome for the particular individual, it needs to be seen in the context of public protection.

References

Bensfield, L.A., Olech, M.J. & Horsley, T.L. (2012) Simulation for high-stakes evaluation in nursing. *Nurse Educator.* **37** (2), 71–4.

Brownie, S., Bahnisch, M. & Thomas, J. (2011). Exploring the literature: Competency-based education and competency-based career frameworks: Deliverable fulfilling part of the requirements for NHPRC Projects 4 and 5 regarding frameworks for competency-based education, training and health career frameworks. University of Queensland Node of the Australian Health Workforce Institute in partnership with Health Workforce Australia, Adelaide, Australia: Australian Health Workforce Institute.

Gaba, D., Howard., S.K., Flanagan, B., Smith, B.E., Fish, K.J. & Botney, R. (1998). Assessment of clinical performance during simulated crises using both technical and behavioural ratings. *Anesthesiology.* **89**, 8–18.

Holmboe, E., Rizzolo, M.A., Sachdeva, A.K., Rosenberg, M. & Ziv, A. (2011). Simulation-based assessment and the regulation of healthcare professionals. *Simulation in Healthcare.* **6** (7), S58–S62.

Kak, N., Burkhalter, B. & Cooper, M-A. (2001). Measuring the competence of healthcare providers. Operations Research Issue Paper 2 (1). Bethesda, MD: Quality assurance (QA) Project.

McKinley, R.K., Strand, J., Ward, L., Gray, T., Alun-Jones, T. & Miller, H. (2008). Checklists for assessment and certification of clinical procedural skills omit essential competencies: a systematic review. *Medical Education.* **42**, 338–49.

Murray, D.J., Boulet, J.R., Kras, J.F., Woodhouse, J.A., Cox, T., and McAllister, J.D. (2004). Acute care skills in anesthesia practice. A simulation-based resident performance assessment. *Anesthesiology.* **101**, 1084–95.

Watterson, L. (2008). Simulation in high-stakes performance assessment, in R.H. Riley (ed.) *Manual of Simulation in Healthcare.* Oxford: Oxford University Press.

Weller, J.M., Bloch, M., Young, S., Maze., M., Oyesola, S., Wyner, J., Dob, D., Haire, K., Durbridge, J., Walker, T. & Newble, D. (2003). Evaluation of high fidelity patient simulator in assessment of performance of anaesthetists. *British Journal of Anaesthesia*. **90** (1), 43–47.

Wolf, L., Dion, K., Lamoureaux, E., Kenny, C., Curnin, M., Hogan, M.A., Roche, J. & Cunningham, H. (2011). Using simulated clinical scenarios to evaluate student performance. *Nurse Educator*. **36** (3), 128–34.

Chapter 12

Quality assurance

Key points

- Quality assurance (QA) should be embedded in the simulation process
- The Department of Health TEL framework provides a useful starting point for QA
- There is a lack of standards for simulation education
- A specific group, with board-level membership, should oversee all simulation activity
- Different professional groups may have different QA requirements

Quality assurance (QA) is described as 'the process for checking that the standards and quality of higher education provision meet agreed expectations' (QAA 2012). Within a university setting, the QA process will be embedded in the curriculum design, faculty development, course evaluation and university management processes, as well as external quality assessment from different agencies and stakeholders. If there is any element of summative assessment, the quality assurance process will also be required to examine its validity and reliability (as discussed in Chapter 11) and standardise it across different sites and with different faculty members.

Within healthcare, there is currently a lack of national in-depth guidance and standards for simulation education (Cummin *et al.* 2008, Weller *et al.* 2012) and so it is difficult to standardise delivery and assess instructor competence (McGaghie *et al.* 2010). Internationally, organisations have started to develop standards and processes such as the accreditation process of the Society of Simulation in Healthcare in North America. However, in the UK at present, anyone can potentially run a simulation session or programme or set up a centre. Whilst the majority of simulation providers are enthusiastic and often experienced clinical experts, they sometimes lack a specific appreciation of how to construct and facilitate sessions. Moreover, as there are no standards of practice, sessions can be run and debriefed in many different ways. This leads to a lack of standardisation of simulation practices, which only increases confusion about simulation terms and expectations, and makes formal research problematic as it is difficult to compare very different programmes. Weller and her colleagues state that the three elements required for an effective simulation-based education programme are infrastructure, curricular integration and trained personnel (Weller *et al.* 2012).

There has been some movement in a positive direction with the recent release of the DH framework for Technology Enhanced Learning (TEL) (DH 2011). This phrase covers various educational activities, including simulation and e-learning, and provides broad, generic guidance on how to deliver a quality, patient-focused, educationally robust event.

As already mentioned, simulation in a non-clinical area will normally have a local educational governance group with an identified lead, whose roles will include quality assurance, ensuring equity of access and business planning. This group will be required to sign off scenarios and programmes and write local policies. It is essential that there is both organisational strategic-level support and also educational support, often through collaboration with local higher education institutions (HEIs). The individual working on their own, developing simulation locally, will often have less time and working knowledge of education governance and local quality assurance process and should therefore be supported by the organisation-based simulation or learning group. Such support may include providing validated scenarios, encouraging relevant local faculty development and assisting in meeting organisational standards.

If learners on a formal academic course are in practice, their academic institution's quality assurance processes may also cover such activities, especially where they are a formal part of the curriculum. Often local lecturers may assist in these sessions, supporting the simulation and practice placement staff. One problem that may arise is when learners from a number of different HEIs, trusts or deaneries participate in a session together. In this situation, there may be a number of different embedded QA processes. It is therefore best to develop a robust quality assurance process that fulfils the various different stakeholder requirements. The QAA has developed a UK quality code for higher education, and the key values of the code (shown below) provide a useful point of reference for simulated learning practices.

Key values of the quality code

- **Students are treated fairly, equitably and as individuals**
- **Students have the opportunity to contribute to the shaping of their learning experience**
- **Students are properly and actively informed at appropriate times of matters relevant to their programmes of study**
- **All policies and processes relating to study are clear and transparent**
- **Strategic oversight of academic standards and academic quality is at the highest level of academic governance**
- **All policies and processes are regularly and effectively monitored, reviewed and improved**
- **Sufficient and appropriate external involvement exists for the maintenance of academic standards and the quality of learning opportunities**
- **Staff are supported, enabling them in turn to support students' learning experiences.**

(QAA 2012)

Putting QA into practice

Once the baseline requirements have been identified, they need to be incorporated into practice. However, rather than seeing this as an onerous task, it can be viewed as a useful process to further the practice of the educator and the course or programme. Research and the QA process can work symbiotically as QA will encourage research, while research data will provide data and evidence for the quality assurance process. Also, as mentioned earlier, clinical governance and simulation are good bedfellows because some of the data from simulation events can provide useful information for clinical governance. This is particularly true when there is a reactive element to simulation training – for example, in response to incidents in an organisation, or in order to prevent incidents by detecting latent errors. Indeed, simple statistics (such as the number of sessions run on a particular ward following an incident) can help demonstrate improvements since the incident.

The following list summarises some of the elements of a well-functioning QA process:

- **Scenarios** – evidence-based, validated, mapped to learners and organisational need
- **Evaluation** – clear evaluation procedure
- **Faculty** – trained, experienced and faculty development encouraged/ routine
- **Learners** – involved in development of programmes and any grievance processes
- **Management** – number of sessions recorded, equipment recorded and maintained, management group with board-level input, relevant standards and policies in place, clear mission statement of simulation, regular review of policies
- **Research** – encouraged
- **External validation by peers and other bodies** – encouraged.

The good news is that the QA process can largely be accomplished automatically if the course/session is constructed in an educationally sound manner, with evaluation embedded throughout its development. There may be times where some of the above points are more aspirational than instantly achievable, especially where an individual is mainly working single-handed. However, the importance of best evidence scenario design, effective debriefing and evaluation cannot be overstated.

Table 12.1: **Putting the QA process into practice**

	Simulation practical elements			
	Scenario development	**Evaluation process**	**Faculty development**	**Management process of education delivery**
Be patient centred and service driven	Clear need for scenario	May include patient groups; improvement measured		Pro-active and reactive
Be educationally coherent	Justifies use of simulation; uses proven education methods for delivery and debriefing	Reviews the educational process as well	Faculty development utilises sound educational process and academic support	Recognises value of evaluation and faculty development
Be innovative and evidence based	Peer reviewed; proven delivery and development process	Use of higher levels of evaluation	Support peer review	Documentation demonstrating course design and validation
Deliver high quality educational outcomes	Embedded relevant learning outcomes, using appropriate simulation delivery and debriefing	Provides evidence of effectiveness	Audit, assessment of faculty development, peer review encouraged, reflection of debriefing	Whole process is aligned to improve patient safety and develop quality learning events
Deliver value for money	Can demonstrate effectiveness	Presentation of numbers trained; demonstrating reducing litigation costs	Internal versus external faculty training	Constant monitoring of throughput, number of sessions and effectiveness
Ensure equity of access and quality of provision	Multi-professional sessions; all staff groups involved	Audits access	All faculty have access; multi-professional faculty	Continuous review of engagement of staff groups

Table 12.1 demonstrates how these six principles can be accomplished in practice and how QA activities can be aligned to the DH framework (DH 2011).

Scenario development

As has already been described in Chapter 2, it is part of the quality assurance process to develop a validated scenario that is fit for purpose, patient centred and evidence based.

The evaluation process

Evaluation of a learning event is sound educational practice, which demonstrates educational coherence and allows both the session and the facilitator to evolve. It is also a way of proving to stakeholders and budget-holders that their money is being wisely and appropriately spent. In effect, we need to embed a quality assurance process within the training from the outset.

There are various ways to evaluate either a single event or programme but evaluation should be a fundamental component in constructing the learning event, and consideration should be given to what and how we are going to evaluate during the session development. It is often useful to audit some of the evaluation areas before the session starts, as this will provide a method of recording the effect of the education session. A thorough evaluation of a learning event will include feedback using various measurement tools, and also a verbal description of the number of sessions, candidates, etc. It is important that these tools show construct validity (i.e. measure what we want to know about). For instance, measuring attendance rate may be useful as part of the evaluation but does not assess the degree of learning that has occurred.

During the session itself, the facilitator carries out continuous evaluation, watching the reaction of the learners, looking for spoken and unspoken clues as to their degree of buy-in, enjoyment and satisfaction. It is possible to evaluate the candidates' learning – although in a subjective non-scientific manner – by seeing them progress and reflect as the session proceeds. Such continuous evaluation allows quieter, nervous or confused learners to be supported, and any issues to be addressed and ideally resolved instantly. Feedback from the learners is also obtained as part of the debriefing session. Asking open-ended questions about what they were feeling and thinking can reveal not only their degree of engagement with the session but also whether or not the underlying educational outcomes are receiving attention. Often, this feedback is not formally recorded. When several facilitators are teaching the session, a facilitator feedback form may therefore be useful in order to collate and capture common themes.

The majority of formal learning events incorporate some type of feedback at the end of the session. These forms often utilise a Likert-type scale to score various aspects of the session, along with space for general comments. However, they are generally limited to the learners' confidence in and satisfaction with the session. One of the criticisms of simulation as a learning tool is the lack of higher levels of evaluation and the reliance on scales that focus on participant satisfaction and self-reported improvement in knowledge and performance (Weller *et al.* 2012). This feedback is more useful for evaluating the general mood of the learners and is often chosen because it is easy to administer and is seen as complying with the requirement for evaluation.

Producing this feedback also requires someone to monitor and record it, which can be burdensome for a large teaching session run regularly. Moreover, the resulting data needs to be used for the benefit of the course and the facilitators. If this information is not communicated to the faculty in a timely manner, the benefit will often be lost. Some caution also needs to be exercised with these feedback forms. Typically, the learners enjoy the sessions if you give them a coffee break, appear organised and finish early, whereas a session that is more challenging for the learners may score less well. Previously validated questionnaires can also be used to look at specific elements such as confidence, stress, awareness and other factors. This makes it easier to compare sessions or undertake research.

Higher-level evaluation

Kirkpatrick described four levels of evaluation (Kirkpatrick 1994). The higher the level of evaluation, the greater the indication that learning or behavioural changes have occurred – but also the more demanding and difficult it is to gather the data. There is a lack of the highest-level evaluation for simulation (Weller *et al.* 2012), partly because it is onerous and labour-intensive to perform, and also because it may be impractical or impossible to achieve for every simulation session. What may be achievable, though, is to audit a smaller number of sessions, looking for changes in practice and patient satisfaction as a marker of improvement.

Table 12.2: **Kirkpatrick's four levels of evaluation**

Kirkpatrick's levels of evaluation	**Description**	**Example of assessment processes**
Level 1: Reactions	Whether learners liked the session	Questionnaires
Level 2: Learning	Whether learners learnt from the session	Pass/fail exam, use of observational validated metrics
Level 3: Behaviour	Whether learners' clinical practice altered	Audits, direct observation in practice, use of observational metrics in practice
Level 4: Results	Whether the training affected organisational aims and objectives	Incident audits, patient satisfaction surveys, root cause analysis investigations

Not surprisingly, learner feedback is the lowest level on Kirkpatrick's scale because of its subjective nature. Higher levels of evaluation can be carried out by looking at the pass rates on the course. On sessions with no pass rates, it may be possible to notice a trend in assessments elsewhere – for instance, by looking at pass rates in resuscitation courses, undergraduate or postgraduate courses.

Notice how the highest levels of evaluation relate directly to the DH TEL framework of education being patient centred (DH 2011). These highest levels of evaluation represent evidence of change in practice, and specifically changes that affect direct patient care. Such data is difficult to obtain, especially when performing short discrete learning sessions. However, if a programme is for a large enough sample of staff, it may be possible to look retrospectively at incident/patient harm events and look for impacts. Imagine that we had run a course for all the junior doctors at a particular hospital trust. The course included, as one of its learning outcomes, clarifying a safe approach to administering IV analgesia. Once all the doctors have been trained, we could look at the number of recorded cases of respiratory depression, ward use of naloxone, or calls involving respiratory arrest to the cardiac arrest team during a month, and compare this data to that from a month before the session was run. From a statistics point of view, the rarer the case, the more difficult it will be to prove a statistically significant change. Specific timings used will depend on local demographics, and observed changes may also depend on other factors. Longitudinal feedback from the learners can also be sought in this case, perhaps asking them direct questions such as 'has the training prevented you from making mistakes with opiates in practice?'

We can also incorporate into evaluation the results from any metrics used as part of the session assessment process, when gathering information for the debriefing. For instance, using a validated tool, we may be able to state that initially 80% of the team could not communicate effectively and this was reduced to 2%, following the session. Although this information is gathered during the simulated event debriefing (rather than in practice), it is still more useful than a simple confidence or satisfaction scale.

Revisiting the programme

Most learning programmes will evolve over time. The facilitators will fine-tune the programme and scenarios, learning from the responses of each group of candidates. Underpinning knowledge may change, reflecting the latest procedures and policies, and this may also require minor changes to the scenarios. This process of evolution is both natural and positive. Formally, once a year, or more often if required by local alterations, there should be an evaluation of the session and a more thorough revisiting should occur, making sure that it is all fit for purpose, there have been no major changes in the subject matter, local guidelines, or learners' curriculum or needs. Ideally, this process should be documented, with a clear paper trail as a form of evidence (if required) for quality assurance. Just as the programme is reviewed on a regular basis, all the management policies and procedures should also be scrutinised regularly. This includes documents pertaining to confidentiality, consent, dealing with learners in difficulty, equality and diversity, and health and safety.

Faculty development

Faculty development clearly does not occur in isolation but needs to be embedded within the training. Evaluation provides rich information on the effectiveness of a learning event, and reflection can enable faculty members to evolve. The faculty needs training and mentoring to develop simulation skills. This will often include faculty development through training, as well as attending national meetings and conferences. This process needs to be continuous, and the faculty's development should be supported and encouraged by management through regular performance reviews and learning needs analysis. There should also be a formal, transparent, statement of the standards and competencies required by the faculty members so that development plans can be made.

For the simulation faculty to remain credible, they need to be up to date with the relevant training (whether it's on resuscitation or another area), and they should be aware of all local relevant clinical skill policies. The simulation faculty can often help to support clinical skills training and it is to be hoped that, in return, staff from these areas will support relevant simulation initiatives. Faculty should also be encouraged to obtain formal academic teaching, simulation and research qualifications, as these can all help to raise the standards of simulation in practice.

Peer review

Peer review of sessions can be useful, both in terms of scenario content and also for the facilitation of the learners. These peer reviews can ideally be documented and retained. Some institutions record the debriefing stage of the event for the faculty to self-reflect, peer review or more formally rate, as a method of faculty development. Building working relationships with facilitators who run similar sessions in neighbouring institutions can also be helpful as a way to further share ideas and best practice.

References

Cummin, D., Merry, A.F. & Weller, J.M. (2008). Standards for simulation. Editorial. *Anaesthesia*. **63**, 1281–4.

Department of Health (2011). *A Framework for Technology Enhanced Learning*. London: HMSO.

Kirkpatrick, D.L. (1994). *Evaluating Training Programs: The Four Levels*. San Francisco, USA: Berrett-Koehler.

McGaghie, W.C., Issenberg, S.B., Petrusa, E.R. & Scalese, R.J. (2010). A critical review of simulation-based medical education research: 2003–2009. *Medical Education*. **44**, 50–63.

QAA (2012). *The UK Quality Code for Higher Education: A Brief Guide*. Gloucester: The Quality Assurance Agency for Higher Education.

Weller, J.M., Nestel, D., Marshall, S.D., Brooks, P.M. & Conn, J.J. (2012) Simulation in clinical teaching and learning. *Medical Journal Australia*. **196** (9), 1–5.

Chapter 13

Example scenario

Title

Anaphylaxis

Overview of the scenario

This scenario focuses on managing the deteriorating patient with an anaphylactic reaction, and initial recognition and management.

Learning outcomes

Respond and assess the deteriorating patient appropriately
Manage anaphylaxis appropriately
Communicate effectively in emergency situations

Equipment needed:

- Manikin with IV access
- Device to simulate rash on manikin
- Drug chart (with recent dose of IV antibiotics noted)
- Notes

- Red allergy wristband
- Emergency trolley with defibrillator
- Adrenaline 1:1000 available (as per trust policy)
- Anaphylaxis algorithm
- 12 Lead ECG (sinus tachycardia)
- Recent blood results (consistent with cellulitis)
- ABG results (acutely hypoxic)

Assessment tools/process (needs knowledge of scope of practice of candidates):

- Copy of Resuscitation Councils Anaphylaxis algorithm as technical skills framework
- Copy of suitable communication part of non-technical skills framework

Expected constitution of learner group (maximum size of 6)

Initial attendance (2 of):
Student nurse, junior nurse, junior physiotherapist, medical student

Local help:
Senior nurse, junior doctor, final year medical student

Response team:
Mid-grade doctor, senior doctor, outreach nurse, night nurse practitioner

Setting the scene

Mary has been admitted with cellulitis (change for context of group as necessary). She has just received her first dose of antibiotics and is complaining of difficulty in breathing.

Initial observations (before starting the scenario)

A: Clear

B: Rapid – 26, wheeze, SaO_2 – 88% (on room air)

C: Pulse 123, BP 90/60, radial pulse present, CRT >3s

D: Alert but distressed

E: Rash

Immediate actions expected from the initially attending staff

- Initiate appropriate assessment – call for help; if help is not requested cue
- Help not available until ABC ascertained – cue learners through ABC
- Hand over to local help when they attend – do not cue handover

Local help attends and finds the following:

1 Clear but facilitator suggests some swelling of lips

2 RR – 28, wheeze SaO_2 – 84% (if on room air), 92% if on high flow oxygen

3 Pulse 135, BP 80/50, no radial pulse, CRT >4s

4 Responding to voice

5 Rash

Expected actions:

- Oxygen – Drop SaO_2 if no supplemental oxygen
- IV fluids – Do not cue
- Call for help (appropriate) – Cue
- Consider anaphylaxis – Do not cue
- Establish cardiac monitoring – Do not cue
- Lead team – Do not cue
- Hand over to senior help (SBAR) – Do not cue

Senior help attends and finds the following:

1 Stridor

2 RR-30, wheeze, SaO_2 – 88% on high flow oxygen

3 Pulse 138, BP 78/47, no radial pulse, CRT>4s

4 Responding to voice/pain

5 Rash

Expected actions:

- Reassess – Do not cue
- Recognises life-threatening anaphylaxis – Cue if not moving forward
- IM adrenaline – Cue use of anaphylaxis emergency algorithm if not moving forward
- Call for senior airway assistance (if not done)
- Reassess – Do not cue
- Lead team – Do not cue
- Communicate treatment plans and 'what if' scenarios – Do not cue
- If not already implemented, connect cardiac monitoring/defibrillator – Do not cue

Patient responds to treatment

Observations:

A: Clear

B: RR-24, SaO_2 97%

C: Pulse 112, BP 127/78, radial pulse present

D: Alert, distressed/emotional

E: Rash fading

Expected actions:

- Reassess – Do not cue
- Confirm senior help on route
- Fluids – Do not cue
- Consider hydrocortisone and chlorphenamine – Do not cue

- Consider transfer for observation to critical care area – Do not cue
- Relevant tests – Do not cue
- Documentation (including drug chart) and cancel antibiotic prescription – Do not cue

Pre-determined debriefing points (to be supplemented by those arising from scenario)

- Use of the available anaphylaxis algorithm to guide treatment
- Location of 1:1000 adrenaline (previous incident – governance request)
- Importance of the rapid administration of IM adrenaline and correct dose
- Communication during the handovers, effective use of SBAR

Educational underpinning material

DH (2009). Competencies for recognising and responding to acutely ill patients in hospital.

NICE (2007). Acutely ill patients in hospital: Recognition of and response to acute illness in adults in hospital. NICE clinical guideline 50.

NICE (2011). Anaphylaxis: assessment to confirm an anaphylactic episode and the decision to refer after emergency treatment for a suspected anaphylactic episode. NICE clinical guideline 134.

Resuscitation Council (UK) (2008). Emergency treatment of anaphylactic reactions. Guidelines for healthcare providers.

Resuscitation Council (UK) (2012). Advanced Life Support Manual.

Trust IV Drug Administration Policy.

Trust Emergency Procedures.

Scenario created by:

Mark Hellaby . . . . Role – Simulation Facilitator

Date:

Validated by:

1) Ian Dillon . . . . Role – ER Charge Nurse

2) Thomas Embry . . . . Role – Senior Resuscitation Officer

Date:

Reviewed by:

1) Claire Brooker . . . . Role – ER Consultant

2) David Tasker . . . . Role – Chair Resuscitation Committee

Date:

Next review planned (may be sooner if policies or procedures change), 12 months from last review.

Date:

Index